A Milieu Therapy Program
for
Behaviorally Disturbed Children

A Milieu Therapy Program
for
Behaviorally Disturbed Children

By

MARJORIE McQUEEN MONKMAN

Associate Professor
Jane Addams Graduate School of Social Work
University of Illinois
Urbana, Illinois

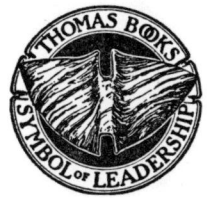

CHARLES C THOMAS • PUBLISHER
Springfield • Illinois • U.S.A.

Published and Distributed Throughout the World by
CHARLES C THOMAS • PUBLISHER
BANNERSTONE HOUSE
301-327 East Lawrence Avenue, Springfield, Illinois, U.S.A.

This book is protected by copyright. No part of it may be reproduced in any manner without written permission from the publisher.

© *1972,* by CHARLES C THOMAS • PUBLISHER
ISBN 0-398-02363-8
Library of Congress Catalog Card Number: 72-184606

With THOMAS BOOKS *careful attention is given to all details of manufacturing and design. It is the Publisher's desire to present books that are satisfactory as to their physical qualities and artistic possibilities and appropriate for their particular use.* **THOMAS BOOKS** *will be true to those laws of quality that assure a good name and good will.*

Printed in the United States of America

For my children
Cindy, Kathy and Johnny

PREFACE

THE STUDY DESCRIBED HERE was supported by the Illinois Research and Training Authority by a grant to Drs. John S. Werry and Marjorie McQueen Monkman and by a U.S. Public Health Service grant number MH 07346 from the National Institute of Mental Health for the period from February, 1967, to July, 1970. Dr. Werry was with the research project from February, 1967, until October, 1968, and his contributions to the program were many.

The success of this research project was accomplished through the efforts of a great many people. As Project Director, I wish to acknowledge the assistance and cooperation of Dr. Robert L. Sprague, Director of the Children's Research Center of the University of Illinois, whose support and encouragement has been very meaningful to me. Dr. William H. Hurder, Mr. Robert L. Harden, and Dr. J. Gregory Langan have all served in the role of Superintendent of the Adler Zone Center during this project. Without the cooperation of these administrators, this project would not have been possible. Mr. Robert L. Symmonds, Unit Manager in charge of Intramural Programs, and Mr. Ronald E. Dolgin, Assistant Superintendent in charge of Extramural Programs, were available to assist me in the many administrative aspects of the project.

I would like to express my warmest thanks to Dr. Elizabeth McInnis who served as Project Coordinator from October 1, 1969. She made valuable contributions to the daily operation of the research project and to the data collection process. She made major contributions to the written description of these operations in Chapters 6 and 7. Dr. McInnis made the major contribution to the development of the punishment study and Chapter 8 is her report of this study. In addition to her research contributions, her relationship with the staff and children helped greatly to develop and maintain a satisfying working and living climate on the cottage.

My thanks go to the six psychology research assistants who have been a part of this research project. David Kuypers and Michael Evans made valuable contributions to the original framework that was used to begin the project. Russell Loo and Roger Bufford were active in the revision of the reinforcement procedures and in the revisions in the data collection process. Joel Match and James Knipe assisted in the final aspects of the project, including the follow-up study. Marian McDonald, a student in psychology, and Russell Loo also made valuable contributions to the pilot follow-up study. In addition to Russell Loo's contributions as a Research Assistant, he served as Cottage Director for a period of six months and made numerous contributions to data analysis processes.

Melvin Hoffman served as Cottage Director from July, 1968, until August, 1969. While in this capacity, he made valuable contributions to the revisions in the project and to the development of the punishment study.

Esther Williams was a part-time research assistant for the duration of the project. Her contributions were many. She did computer programming for the entire project. She was readily available for assistance in data analysis and willingly transported research-project data to and from the Digital Computer Laboratory, University of Illinois.

Freida Carpenter, Sandra O'Meara, Carolyn Kemp, and Leonard Kemp were social work students who served their field experience from June, 1969, to February, 1970, under the supervision of the Project Director. These four students contributed greatly to the development and implementation of the home programs for the children who were in residence at the cottage during this period.

I wish to express deep appreciation to the child-care staff, teachers, and Extramural Case Coordinators, who gave thoughtful service to the children in this project and feedback to the project staff that made possible the constant development of this research project.

Finally, I wish to thank Mrs. Lois Haig for her editorial assistance in the preparation of this report. As we worked together over the successive drafts, Mrs. Haig helped me to express essential ideas and to present them in a meaningful form and order.

Space does not permit the detailed description of every important change that occurred in the development of this research project. I have, therefore, attempted to present a detailed description of the program as it was at the end of the granting period, to show the process of major changes in the project, and to give some rationale for these decisions. There are still many parts that should be developed. My goal is not to offer a definitive and final statement on the treatment of children, but rather to contribute to the formulation of knowledge in the field.

MARJORIE McQUEEN MONKMAN

CONTENTS

	Page
Preface	vii

Chapter
1. INTRODUCTION TO THE RESEARCH PROJECT 3
2. THE MILIEU 12
   Dimension 1 14
   Dimension 2 16
   Dimension 3 17
   Dimension 4 18
   Dimension 5 20
3. THE CHILD AND THE TREATMENT PROCESS 33
4. INSTRUMENTS FOR RESEARCH-PROJECT EVALUATION 38
5. CHILD-CARE TRAINING FOR RESEARCH-PROJECT STAFF 50
6. IMPLEMENTATION OF THE MILIEU PROGRAM 62
7. INDIVIDUAL PROGRAMS 84
   Subject 10 84
   Subject 19 90
   Subject 21 101
8. PUNISHMENT STUDY 113
9. ASSESSMENT OF THE RESEARCH PROJECT 125

References 135

Appendices
A. DESCRIPTION OF STAFF ROLES 139
B. INSTRUMENT SAMPLES 145
C. PROCEDURES AND POLICIES 173
D. SUPPLEMENTAL INFORMATION FOR ONE INDIVIDUAL PROGRAM .. 197

E. PROGRAMS FOR TWENTY-SEVEN CHILDREN 221
F. SAMPLES OF INSTRUMENTS USED IN FOLLOW-UP STUDY 273

Index 283

A Milieu Therapy Program
for
Behaviorally Disturbed Children

Chapter 1

INTRODUCTION TO THE RESEARCH PROJECT

THE NEED FOR RESEARCH in ongoing practice situations has been recognized for some time. The vast number of interacting variables in practice situations have made research very difficult. A number of major variables are important at any one point in time; however, control of any major variable is hard. The fact that many important variables have to be manipulated simultaneously has made the ongoing practice situation less apt to encourage research than the laboratory or a controlled experimental condition. The time to move research into the practice situation is well past, and the need is urgent.

It was for this reason that the Children's Research Center of the University of Illinois was situated near the Herman M. Adler Zone Center of the Illinois Department of Mental Health. An area map (Fig. 1) indicates the proximity of the physical facilities of the Children's Research Center and the Adler Zone Center. This complex is located in the southern part of the University of Illinois campus at Urbana-Champaign. It was envisioned that the Children's Research Center would inaugurate and facilitate programs of research in the Adler Zone Center, which is the headquarters for the Illinois Department of Mental Health's program for children and adolescents in Zone 6, covering eighteen counties in East Central Illinois and serving over a quarter-million children.

This research project was the first such major venture. The project was given program jurisdiction over the Adler Zone Center's Cottage G, one of three residential cottages that provide training and treatment for a total of 48 mentally retarded and/or emotionally disturbed children. An experimental, residential treatment program was developed.

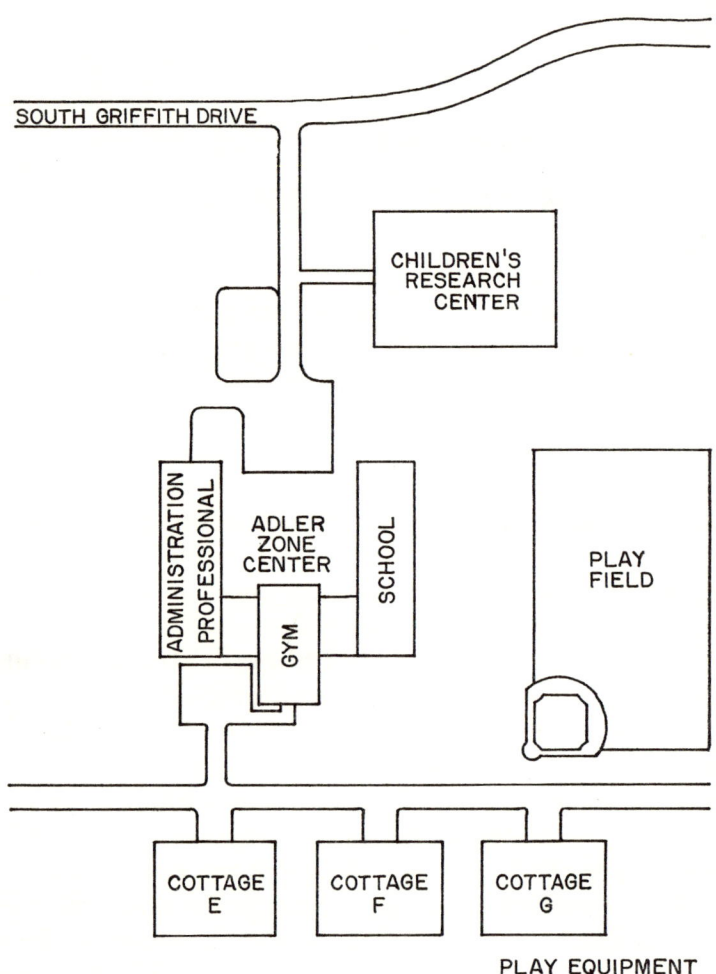

Figure 1. Area map of the Children's Research Center and the Adler Zone Center.

Diligent attention to lines of communication made it possible to operate in a complex situation such as this one, i.e. to operate a clinical service program that afforded opportunities for research. It was essential for the Adler personnel to respect the necessity for research in clinical practice, and for the researchers and academic personnel to respect the necessity for investigating problems that were meaningful to clinicians without contravening the clinical ethnic. Both the researcher and the clinician were interested in showing positive change in the children who were served in the unit. Thus, it was the perspective of this project that the clinical program and the research were not different. The intervention that was carried on by the clinician was the researcher's independent variable.

Goals of the Adler Zone Center

One of the primary goals of the Adler Zone Center is to facilitate the development of comprehensive, community mental health programs for emotionally disturbed and/or mentally retarded children and their families. It is not the purpose of the Adler Zone Center to duplicate existing services, but rather to work with existing resources in assessing community needs and services. The Adler Zone Center hopes to assist communities in developing the services needed to meet the identified needs, and hopes to develop projects that illustrate methods of giving greater service and of enlisting community support.

A second major goal of Adler is to develop services for children that offer "continuity of care," i.e. services that give continuous care to the child and his family from the time the problem comes to the attention of the agency until the child is functioning at maximum capacity in the community.

Another significant goal of the Adler Zone Center is to investigate the methods and results of service for the purpose of adding to the body of knowledge concerning the cause and treatment of emotionally disturbed and/or mentally retarded children.

Goals of the Children's Research Center

The Children's Research Center was established as an interdisciplinary research center with two major goals:

1. To do research on the remediation of emotionally disturbed and/or mentally retarded children.
2. To do research on the training of mental health personnel.

The major focus of the Children's Research Center is the development of basic knowledge of remediation of emotionally disturbed and/or mentally retarded children, which could be used to train mental health personnel.

Goals of the Research Project

The first major goal of the research project was that of conceptualizing an ongoing service program in such a manner that the crucial therapeutic variables could be identified, taught, replicated, and evaluated. Thus, this research project was seen as a process study rather than an outcome study. It was evident that it was not possible to measure the outcome until the variables that were being manipulated in the program were clearly identified and described.

A second goal was to develop techniques to be used by the child-care staff in direct interaction with the children, and to specify attitudes and behaviors that were useful in the day-to-day interactions between the child-care staff and the individual child.

A third goal of the project was to develop a curriculum for training all staff who were directly involved in the treatment programs. Both the content of the treatment programs and the methods employed to teach this content were considered important aspects of the project.

A fourth goal was to establish a set of clinically acceptable criteria for progress of the children who were served in the project and to develop instruments for effectively measuring these changes.

A fifth goal was to offer learning opportunities to University of Illinois students and to Adler personnel who were interested in the rehabilitation of behaviorally disturbed children.

The final and much valued goal of the program was to develop and to operate an effective program that produced significant and lasting changes of its residents, in the direction of better social adaptation and in a manner that was consonant with the ethical standards of society in general. By so doing, it was hoped that the capacity of the individuals would be enhanced and that they would achieve greater human realization.

Administrative Arrangements and Staffing

Administrative lines of authority and cooperation for the research project were complex, owing to the involvement of both the Adler Zone Center of the Illinois Department of Mental Health and the Children's Research Center of the University of Illinois (Fig. 2). It was obvious that for reasons of sheer practicality and efficiency, the operating authority of the project had to reside in one person. Thus, the responsibility for administering the research project in Adler was that of the Project Director from the Children's Research Center. The Project Director was subject only to the veto of the Director of the Children's Research Center and the Superintendent of the Adler Zone Center.

The Project Director made decisions on matters of operating policy and research; supervised directly the Project Coordinator, Cottage Director, Project Secretary, research assistants, and the independent observers; and supervised indirectly the child-care workers. The Cottage Director had direct supervision over the child-care workers. The three state civil-service classifications for the workers were Mental Health Worker, which required a college degree; Mental Health Program Assistant, which required at least two years of college; and Child Care Aide, which required a high school degree.

Staff classified as Mental Health Workers were assigned to be Intramural Counselors to the individual child. Other child-care workers were designated as Assistant Counselors. Appendix A lists the duties and responsibilities of the Intramural Counselor and also those of the Project Coordinator, the Cottage Director, and the Extramural Case Coordinator, who was a professional staff member (psychiatrist, psychologist, social worker, etc.) employed in the extramural division of the Adler Zone Center.

The Project Director, Project Coordinator, research assistants, Project Secretary, and independent observers were employed from research grant funds; the direct-service personnel of Cottage G, Cottage Director, and child-care workers were employed by the Adler Zone Center.

There was a rapid turnover of staff since students from the

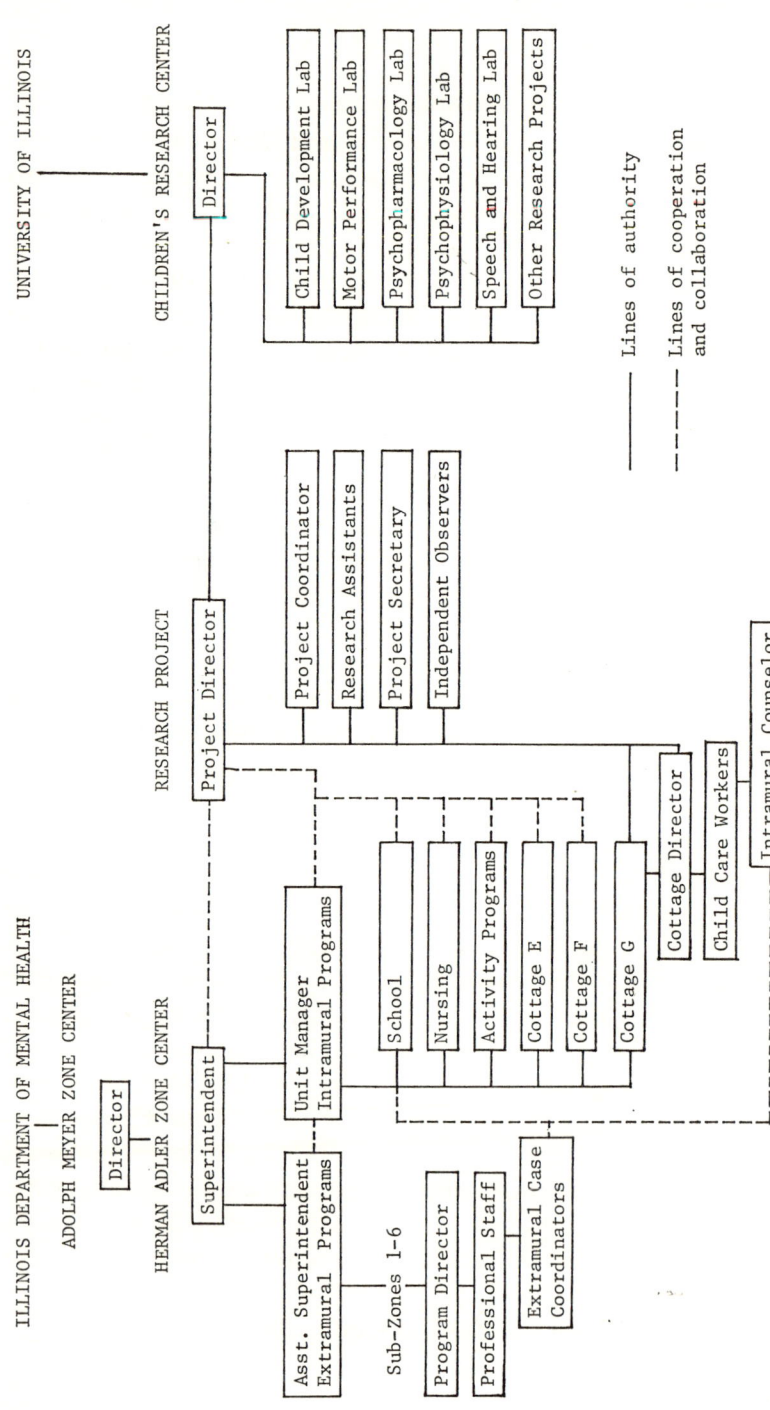

Figure 2. Organizational Chart showing lines of authority and cooperation within the research project.

University of Illinois were used as research assistants and independent observers, and students or their spouses made up most of the child-care workers. In the two and one-half years during which the research project operated the unit, only four child-care workers, from a total of 38, were with the project from the beginning; in addition, there were three different cottage directors.

The Project Coordinator, who was with the project for 20 months, contributed considerably to continuity. It was recognized that individual skills of workers affected considerably, at any one point in time, the operation of the unit and the services given to a child. The enthusiasm of the staff maintained an atmosphere that contributed to the success of the research project. The rapid turnover in staff, however, shows that the operation of the unit was not maintained because of the functioning of any individual child-care worker but, more important, was maintained because of the conceptualization and overall operation of the research design.

Admission Procedures

In keeping with the Adler policy of being a short-term facility with a maximum stay of one year, the major criteria for admission to Adler Zone Center are (a) that the child can benefit within one year from the available Adler residential programs and (b) that the child will return to the family and community upon discharge. If the child cannot return to the family, Adler's extramural staff works with the family and appropriate agencies to develop a program for alternative placement. The admission of children who are clearly in need of custodial or indefinitely long care and treatment would be an unwise use of this resource; therefore, the intramural program does not offer custodial treatment, and beds are not available for detention. It should be noted that children whose needs are primarily medical cannot be admitted, as sophisticated medical facilities and services are not available at Adler.

Cases identified by a community agency as requiring residential treatment are referred to the Adler extramural staff for evaluation. The Adler staff investigates the case and makes some decision regarding whether it is appropriate for outpatient or residential care. If they feel it is an appropriate case for short-term residential care, they contact the director of one of the cottages and discuss the case with him. If he agrees that it sounds like a potential residential case, then a preadmission meeting is scheduled to make the formal decision to accept the child for residential treatment.

For admission to the research-project cottage, the people at the preadmission meetings included the Cottage Director, the Extramural Case Coordinator requesting the admission, the Program Director from the subzone involved, a teacher from the Adler school, and a representative from the referring community agency. While either the Project Director or Project Coordinator usually attended these meetings, they were there as nonvoting observers. Thus, the decision to accept or not accept a child for admission to the research project was made by those representing the Adler Zone Center. For admission to the research-project cottage, the only modifications of the Adler criteria were some restrictions, established by project personnel, regarding the children's level of functioning and age.

Six weeks after admission, each case was reviewed by Adler's Clinical Review Committee, which was composed of three intramural and three extramural staff members, and a discharge date was agreed upon. The child's treatment program, the child's progress in his program, and the plans and implementation of plans for the child's discharge were reviewed periodically during the child's stay at Adler. By design, the research project for Cottage G required an initial period of three months in order to assess adequately the child's adjustment to the program. Children in Cottage G were reviewed at six weeks, but minimum admission was for three months; however, an agreed-upon discharge date was set at the initial clinical review.

The Research - Project Sample

This report describes the treatment of a group of thirty children who were served at various times during the period from February, 1968, to May 1, 1970. From February, 1968, to

February, 1969, eight children were admitted to the residential treatment program and formed the nucleus for developing the program and for training the staff. The group of thirty children ranged in intelligence from high trainable to gifted. Each child admitted to the unit had, within his repertoire, basic self-care skills, i.e. he was basically toilet trained, able to dress and feed himself. Each child had language and understood a minimal amount of language, and no child was severely overtly psychotic, although a number of the children demonstrated bizarre behaviors. The children were between the ages of seven and thirteen.

Framework of the Research Project

During the research project, an effort was made to develop a milieu that offered appropriate opportunities for development to the children. Programs were set up for them that enabled the children to progress toward a desired terminal pattern of behavior. The programs were designed to communicate to the children what was required of them; how they were able to receive positive attention from the staff, privileges and rewards; and how to discriminate between desirable and undesirable behavior.

A framework of five dimensions, which are described in detail in Chapter 2, served as the guidelines for directing action toward the children.

Chapter 2

THE MILIEU

THE TERM "milieu therapy" has become familiar in the helping professions. It is a mode of treatment that recognizes and uses the effects of the environment on the individual condition. The variables of the milieu rarely have been specified or used consistently in the planning of a milieu program.

The general working principle of this research project was that the therapeutic process could be most usefully and heuristically conceptualized within the scientific framework. To apply the principles of science, attention was paid to smaller and smaller elements of the practice situation through the elaboration of constructs and through the development of measuring instruments. The relations between the behavioral acts and the constructs that were used to describe the overall milieu were made as explicit as possible. The pieces or discrete bits of behavior that were used to measure the change in the individual child were specified as clearly as possible. Attention was given to stating the cognitive links between the observable behavior, any references that were made about the variables which affected change in these behaviors, and the content of the milieu that affected the change in the individual behavior.

The milieu of this research project was perceived as a number of processes existing and moving and changing over a period of time. These processes consisted of physical and social variables interacting with each other.

Among all variables, a number of interconnections were postulated. These interconnections represented a flow of influences in the environment. This flow of influences was constructed in such a way that it increased the probability of specified human actions. Thus, it was possible to conceptualize and to develop an ongoing complex of interrelated expectations that were separated from the individual child. The expectations existed in the milieu separate from the individual child, affected the individual child, and in turn were affected by the individual child. They were thought of as requirements and opportunities for the individual child.

In this research project, these variables were referred to as dimensions of the milieu. It is important to state that these dimensions were constructed around the objectives of a treatment program for all children and were not constructed around the problems of the individual child.

Dimensions were defined as conceptual aspects or components of the overall phenomena with which we were dealing. The dimensions were areas or categories of the phenomena, but they were not equal to each other. They were seen as interdependent major forces, which operated in the milieu in a way that guided the actions of those involved in the project. They were not mutually exclusive; they were not all dealing with phenomena at the same level of abstraction; and they were not equally well developed conceptually.

The dimensions of the milieu were as follows:

Dimension 1—a progressive movement system from admission to discharge.
Dimension 2—daily routines and minimum appropriate self-care behaviors.
Dimension 3—categories of expected social functioning.
Dimension 4—a feedback and reinforcement system.
Dimension 5—a punishment system.

These dimensions were used as guidelines to train the staff, to build the content of the program, to specify treatment programs, to direct therapeutic action of the staff, and to develop instruments of measurement for evaluating change in the children.

Each of the dimensions did not make an identical contribution to every facet of the milieu. Dimension 1, a core dimension to which every other dimension related, served as a guideline for the overall treatment objectives of the program, i.e. to return the child to the community with improved ways of coping with the opportunities and demands of his environment. Dimension 2, important in structuring the content of the daily operations, offered a list of expected behaviors to be developed in those children who did not have them, and this list of behaviors served as a measuring instrument for the research project. Dimension 3, a more complex dimension which was less well developed, served (a) as a guideline for categorizing desirable social skills that should be developed in each child; (b) to train staff to think about the areas of social functioning to be developed in each child; and (c) as a beginning guideline to measure increases in social skill. Dimension 3 also affected the content of the milieu curriculum. Dimension 4, a system of feedback and a program of reinforcers, was a major dimension in guiding the action of the staff in relation to the treatment objectives that were guided principally by Dimensions 1, 2, and 3. Dimension 4 emphasized ways of communicating the expectations of the treatment program and of enhancing the level of social functioning of the children. Dimension 5, the most completely developed dimension, indicated for staff and children the undesirable behaviors and the consequences of specific undesirable behaviors. Dimension 5 was used to train staff to deal with these behaviors and as a measure of change for undesirable behavior. The application of these dimensions is discussed more completely in the following description of each dimension.

Dimension 1

The first dimension was a progressive movement system from admission to discharge back into the community. Dimension 1 was considered to be the basic conceptual dimension of the program and overlapped each of the other dimensions.

In order to accomplish the objectives of the program, the system was constructed so that each child was required to engage increasingly in behavior that was appropriate for living in the community. Therefore, a movement system was proposed in which each child was required to progress through a series of levels in the program with each successive level requiring more responsible behavior than the preceding one.

There were a number of basic ideas that were predominant in the movement system from the beginning. One idea was to use concrete reinforcers initially, if necessary, but to move the child off these reinforcers later. A second idea was to have the child spend an increasingly large amount of time in community activities, e.g. in his own home, in the public school, and in community recreational activities. A third idea was to enable the child to have more appropriate control of his behavior so that the already built-in standards and expectations of the community would sustain the behavior in the child adequately when he returned to the community.

The progressive movement system had an entrance level (orientation) and three treatment levels (I, II, and III).

Orientation Level

Before a more structured approach to his activities was begun, the Orientation Level demonstrated what the child would do in a situation when it was less structured. On the Orientation Level, reinforcers were given noncontingently, i.e. activities, treats, etc., were given freely whether or not individual behavior warranted them. Only grossly undesirable behavior was punished. The child was given the opportunity to do the expected self-care and household tasks, but specific contingencies were not applied to this behavior.

In the progressive movement system, it was important that the entrance level should allow for immediate achievement. To see achievement was important both to the child and to the staff. A very exciting part of implementing the progressive movement system was the fact that a child, when put on the Orientation Level where everything was noncontingent, very often became motivated to receive a program in order to begin to work on skills that he needed to develop in himself and to work on undesirable behaviors that he was emitting on the unit.

Level I

This first treatment level of the progressive movement system contained the first behaviors that were to be used as targets in the child's program. These usually were concrete kinds of behaviors and were already in the child's repertoire of behaviors.

Perhaps the child was taught to respond initially to the contingencies rather than to learn a new behavior, i.e. getting him "hooked" on the system.

Level II

On this treatment level, the behaviors that were labeled as targets for change usually were more complex and represented the kind of change that would enable the child to adapt better to his home, school, and community situations. Because of the complexity of these behaviors, Level II was constructed with sublevels that were identified as Phases I, II, III, and IV. The number of phases used for a Level II program varied for each child with the number and complexity of the targets. These targets were stated in prosocial terms and were behaviors in which an increase in quantity and often in quality were desirable. They were behaviors with which reinforcers (Dimension 3) were paired.

Level III

This level of the movement system was thought of as a reorienting level. The focus was on developing the child's community program. The behavior targets were those that were most relevant to his home, school, and community situations. The contingencies were those items and social attitudes that were available to him in the community or that could be made available through more appropriate use of normative community resources.

Dimension 2

The second dimension consisted of the daily routines and the minimum appropriate self-care behaviors expected of each child living in the cottage. The minimum appropriate behaviors (MAB) were itemized on the Daily Checklist. The Daily Checklist constituted a research instrument that served as a record of whether or not the child performed routine self-care behaviors, including washing hands, showering, brushing teeth, dressing, and getting to meals on time. During the first few weeks on the cottage, the MAB list was used to assess the performance rate of the child on these behaviors. It subsequently served as an index to measure change in the child's performance following the treatment procedure. Thus, Dimension 2 of the milieu and the measurement of the child's performance were directly related. In addition, the child's treatment program, which specified the behaviors that it was desirable to incorporate in him, was directly related to the structure and the measurement of the program. On the cottage, activities were structured around the Daily Checklist in such a way that a certain amount of ritual was created in connection with the behaviors which were related to regular functions, e.g. feeding, going to bed, dressing, taking a bath. Regular times were set aside for these activities and presented the opportunity for these behaviors to occur. Requirements, in relation to these behaviors, were made quite clear, and rewards were offered for the accomplishment of these behaviors.

Dimension 3

The third dimension consisted of categories of expected social functioning, appropriate social behaviors (ASB), to be developed and evaluated for every child. Dimension 3 differed from the second dimension in that Dimension 2 was made up of concrete behaviors that were observable and a part of the daily activities. The categories of appropriate social behaviors were not discrete behaviors, but they represented areas of development for the child's functioning. These categories were operationalized in concrete terms and served as guidelines in developing the program for the individual child. Quality and quantity of the behaviors for each child varied within the individual program.

The various types of appropriate social behaviors were grouped into the following six major categories:

1. Cooperative behavior—self-initiated cooperative behavior on the part of the child, e.g. aiding a staff member in the performance of some task, volunteering to perform a task, etc.

2. Sharing—allowing another child or staff member to use something he has been using or giving an item to another child or staff member—could be upon or without request by the staff member or other child.

3. Helping—giving assistance to another child or staff member, e.g. aiding another child in the performance of some task or game, or helping another child with school work.

4. Participation—taking part in structured activities that were initiated by, and under direct supervision of, a staff member in which the expectancy was that the child would engage in the activity, e.g. listening to a story read by a staff member.

5. Interaction—taking part in unstructured activities, i.e. activities that were self-initiated, which were not organized by the staff and in which participation was not expected, e.g. playing pool with another child, talking with a staff member, greeting visitors.

6. Constructive—self-directed activity aimed at the betterment of the child or constructive use of time in which the child was not interacting or participating with other children or staff members, e.g. reading, writing, watching TV, knitting, building models.

These categories consistently remained as guidelines for the development of the milieu program and for the development of an individual child's treatment program.

Dimension 4

The fourth dimension was a system of feedback and reinforcement. Feedback refers to the consequences of output, i.e. consequences that were fed back into the processing to affect succeeding output. In the context of this dimension, reinforcement was implemented through the deliberate use of a program of reinforcers: A reinforcer was an event or item (such as food, attention, or an opportunity to participate in desired activity) that, when presented to the child following a desirable behavior, was hypothesized to increase the probability that he would behave in that way again in a similar situation. Emphasis was placed on the need for consistency in the feedback system and for flexibility in the program of reinforcers. For this reason, the program of reinforcers is discussed separately.

Feedback System

A system that fed back to the child that his behavior was appropriate was essential to the treatment process. This system had to be constant and consistent. The feedback system was used in relation to the behavioral expectations of the program. Feedback of the desired information was communicated to the child at the appropriate level and took many forms, e.g. verbal and nonverbal behavior of staff and tangible material objects. When each child reached his Level I in the movement system (Dimension 1), he was presented with a Mark Sheet that had his targets of treatment labeled for him. Next to each target were spaces for a staff member to mark when the child emitted a desired behavior. It was uniformly known and constantly communicated in the program that it was appropriate to get marks in all the spaces on your Mark Sheet. This feedback system was deliberately paired with a reinforcer. Although the purpose of the program was to increase desirable behavior, the feedback system also communicated that a specific behavior was inappropriate.

Program of Reinforcers

Reinforcers varied between children and varied with the individual child at different times. The program of reinforcers was kept flexible, novel, idiosyncratic, and timely.

The symbols of social approval (smile, praise, etc.) and backup reinforcers (candy, toys, recreational activities, home visits, etc.) made up the program of reinforcers. The staff gave verbal praise, a smile, and so forth, with the distribution of marks. These marks were exchangeable for backup reinforcers. While the marks themselves fed back to the child that his behavior was desirable to the staff, this information did not necessarily have reinforcing value for the child. In fact, he sometimes was influenced more by staff disapproval. It became very important to pair the message of approval with a powerful tangible reinforcer so that he was motivated more to receive the social reinforcer than he was to receive the disapproval of the adults in his environment. This was one of the first steps in changing the "meaning" of behavior for the child.

The relation of backup reinforcers to social reinforcers also was important since, ultimately, it was expected that much of the behavior would be sustained by social reinforcers. The basis for social reinforcers was that much of the behavior would be sustained through the child's satisfaction in achieving the requirements. With some children, backup reinforcers were used and were paired with social reinforcers in order to make social reinforcers meaningful and, in turn, to make achievement meaningful. Some children found the social reinforcers meaningful from the beginning, and some children even found the social reinforcers more meaningful than the backup.

Thus, experience demonstrated that movement was not necessarily sequential from a backup reinforcer to a social reinforcer for children of this age and with these types of problems.

Dimension 5

The fifth dimension, a system for punishing undesirable behavior, developed over a period of time and was the most completely developed dimension. This dimension labeled and categorized undesirable behavior according to severity and gave explicit direction to staff for interventive action with respect to undesirable behavior. In addition, this dimension was conceptualized in a manner that enabled measurement of the kind and the frequency of undesirable acts. Comparison was made of the effects of two types of punishment, time out and response cost. The time-out procedure used was to remove the child from the ongoing situation and to place him in an isolation room for a certain length of time. The response-cost procedure took the form of fines that the child paid with marks which he earned.

Categories for punishable behavior included the following:

100 Level—defiance of minor rules and requests
                minor-moderate tantrums
                minor-moderate verbal abuse
                minor-moderate physical abuse

200 Level—defiance of more serious rules and requests
                lying
                attempted provocation

300 Level—defiance of major rules and requests
                severe tantrum behavior

The Milieu

       severe verbal abuse
       minor assault (on children)
       attempted framing
       minor destruction of property
       threatening (staff or children)
400 Level—verbal extortion and bribery
       urinating or defecating in an inappropriate place
       leaving the time-out room without permission
       talking to a child who was in time out
       tearing up a door chart
       aiding and abetting another's misbehavior by impeding staff
500 Level—assault (on children)
       forgery
       serious destruction of property
       extortion through use of physical force
       possession of forbidden, harmful, or dangerous items
       stealing
       inappropriate sexual behavior
600 Level—assault (on an adult)
       AWOL
       entering the cottage office
700 Level—self-destructive behavior
       soiling behavior
       idiosyncratic deviant behavior

A study of the effects of time-out and response-cost punishment procedures, using the 100 through 500 Level behaviors, is presented in Chapter 8.

Evolvement of the Dimensions

Each of the dimensions underwent change as a result of experience. The first attempt to accomplish the ideas for progressing through the program was to tie the movement system (Dimension 1) very closely to the reward system (Dimension 4) so that, as time passed, the children would earn rewards that were related more to activities in the community. As a result of this, the measurement scale, objectives, and reinforcement system were confused; consequently, more potent and more numerous reinforcers were too delayed. After experimenting with the reinforcers, it was perceived that a change in the movement system was needed so that it corresponded with the treatment targets; and the program of reinforcers needed to be separate so that it could deal more individually with each child. Thus, the movement system was left as one that set targets for the child to return to the community, but it allowed greater flexibility in the reinforcement system.

In the original progressive movement system, the first level allowed a minimum number of plastic tokens to be earned and allowed a minimum way of spending these on the cottage without opportunities to get off the grounds. It was hoped that the child would earn his way up so that he would have more and greater opportunities over time to participate in things in the community. The result of this seemed to be that a more deviant milieu began to develop since the children were unable to get out of the situation, and the nature of their interactions on the unit reinforced undesirable behavior. However, another result occurred that was positive. This was the fact that the children were together on the unit, and the necessity for dealing with their undesirable interaction on the unit caused the staff to become more creative in on-unit activities and to find more ways of diverting their behavior. These skills probably contributed to the overall program as time passed; whereas, it could be postulated that if the children had been allowed more freedom in participating in outside activities from the very beginning of the program, this would have been used as a way to entertain the children rather than to create more ways of dealing with the children's problems in interaction with each other. Watching this created awareness of the need to offer both kinds of opportunities regularly.

Most of the targets for the children's programs were stated in connection with the dimensions that specified appropriate behaviors (Dimensions 2 and 3). These appropriate behaviors were included in the child's program for progress in such a way as to give him appropriate targets for movement rather than undesirable behaviors or problems as targets for treatment.

In the early stages of the program, some of the MAB Daily Checklist items were tokened, and others were left untokened. The resulting data seemed to show that some items, tokened or not, were done more often by all children. This particularly seemed to be the case if the behavior occurred at a specific time when all children were performing the task in the presence of staff. The frequency of performance seemed related to the ritual associated with the task. A small number of the children seemed to discriminate between tokened and nontokened items; however, some children never seemed to perform some of the specific behaviors, whether tokened or not. This led to making the reinforcers contingent on the neglected behaviors. This usually was included in Level I of the movement system (Dimension 1). Thus, the MAB Daily Checklist (Dimension 2) became one guideline for the treatment programs.

The definitions of the categories of appropriate social behaviors (Dimension 3) changed over a period of time. The emphasis on the categories changed and to some extent, so did the use of the categories. Experience with the six categories, in relation to the cottage, called attention to the future need for two additional categories that would be particularly important for the older children. These categories could be labeled "grooming" and "sex-role behaviors." This latter category was one where the need for developing new behaviors, in addition to teaching the child to use the appropriate behaviors that were already acquired, was indicated. Programs of sex education were needed in the curriculum also.

The ASB dimension, although it was the weakest dimension, was very important to the entire program. It was important because it was the principle dimension used to set up the targets for the individual child's program (Dimension 1, Level II targets). Dimension 3 was weak because it was difficult to conceptualize in operational terms and was not always recognized as a target setting dimension by the staff.

One problem was that individual target setting, i.e. categories of desired behaviors to be developed or encouraged in the child, was confused with setting up the content of the program that would be used as the structure for bringing about change in the child. The curriculum or opportunities for developing these behaviors and the categories of desirable behavior did not specify these differences, and they did not automatically occur together, e.g. the difference between the ASBs and the MABs. The MABs were behaviors that primarily occurred at particular times; therefore, both the curriculum or content of the program and the behavior were specific and closely associated. In the ASB categories, the behaviors were not specific; therefore, curriculum to encourage these behaviors needed to be considered and worked on. This kind of thinking was not incorporated into the overall program as much as would be desired.

The use of the ASBs as target-setting behaviors also differed from the punishment dimension (Dimension 5) because behaviors that were unacceptable were easier for everybody to define. It was never appropriate to hit somebody. The appropriate social behaviors were more qualitative and had to be considered in relation to age, sex, and ability of the individual child. This made the specifying of prosocial behaviors much more qualitative. Many appropriate behaviors were defined in relation to specific situations. There were behaviors that occurred only in a specific situation; and although very desirable in that situation, encouragement was needed in relation to time and place. Thus, the number of aspects that had to be considered in developing the categories of prosocial functioning were complex.

Another problem with the ASBs was that of measurement. In measuring many of the prosocial behaviors that the staff wished to encourage in the children, the measurement of the prosocial behavior needed to relate to the situation in which the behavior occurred. A number of the behaviors, which were quite relevant when they occurred, did not occur with great frequency and more often than not occurred in specific situations so that the measuring instrument needed to be related to those situations. The fact that the behavior occurred infrequently did not mean that the behavior was not very important when it did occur. Adequate and appropriate measuring devices for infrequent specific behaviors were needed in order to show change in them.

Another important aspect of the ASBs was that of communication. Because of qualitative differences in children, i.e. age, sex, ability, a particular behavior was called idiosyncratic for a child. Labeling that behavior as something idiosyncratic did not mean that it did not fit appropriately into a category of behaviors. It was easy to confuse this individual communication system with an individual program. The importance of communication and the idiosyncratic nature of communication was recognized, but the need for categorizing and gaining reliability at higher levels of abstraction across more behaviors had to be recognized by the researcher and by the practitioner also. It has been noted by most practitioners that children tend to have either "good" or "bad" behaviors. Thus, there seemed to be a need to categorize prosocial behaviors that were already in the repertoire of the child differently from those social skills that were undeveloped. Those that were undeveloped needed to be stated as specific targets and to be programmed progressively, while those that were available to the child needed to be reinforced more by an overall target, such as cooperation. There were a few specific targets, such as increasing verbalizations with peers and adults, but many times the targets were to increase the amount of time and the number of activities in which the child chose to use his already established array of prosocial behaviors.

The need for generalizing and for constructing ways of generalizing prosocial behavior was another important aspect. The data showed that it was possible to alter behavior by communicating to the child what the contingencies were for both prosocial and antisocial behavior. Once this was done, the need for generalizing with relation to other situations was apparent immediately. After control of the behavior was gained and the child understood how to produce a more desirable kind of behavior, the need to increase the number of situations in which the prosocial behavior could be used should be planned for immediately. This was an aspect of the developing of targets that was not accomplished as adequately as was desirable.

The staff tended to concretize the ASB categories and made

each category a behavior or a limited number of behaviors. It was difficult for them to deal with both the amount and kind of idiosyncratic behaviors exhibited by the children in relation to each ASB category.

Considering all aspects of the milieu, the dimension that changed the most was the program of reinforcers (Dimension 4). Initially, the program of reinforcers was set up to reinforce each child in almost the same way and with the same materials. The child was given very few privileges, and these were earned by the child over a period of time. With increased good behavior, he gained more and more reinforcers. In addition, the reinforcers were set up so that the child's area of activity expanded as his desirable behavior increased. In the beginning of his program, the child was much more limited in his activities. These activities were all confined to the unit and increased to community activities and privileges as he progressed in his treatment program.

This type of orientation proved to have many problems. One was the delay. Some privileges were too far in the future for some children, particularly the younger children in the program. In addition, some of the privileges that were offered had never been experienced by the child; consequently, they were not motivating to him. Also, reinforcers are idiosyncratic. Some children never were as interested in a particular activity as others were. If reinforcers were going to be used to develop behaviors in children, it was necessary to make them either truly reinforcing or things that the children wanted. The program of reinforcement changed, consequently, to enable the child to use almost any reinforcer from the beginning of his program, and reinforcement was set up so that it could be used quite individually.

There was a project system of reinforcers. A list of activities and concrete materials was available for the staff to use in developing the individual programs. In the beginning, plastic tokens were used for the child to earn his backup reinforcers; and social praise from the staff, along with the tokens, was emphasized. As stated earlier (Dimension 4), the more recent system used a mark, rather than the plastic token, for feedback to the child. One backup for a child was to spend his marks at a store, which was open at certain times of the day. The store contained food, recreational items (such as games, books, and gadgets), and articles for personal care. A game room was available for "rent," and the makeup of the room was altered frequently so that it continued to be a place that the children wished to go. It had, at various times, a juke box, bumper pool, and Ping-Pong table. Cottage parties were a major reinforcer. A regular party was organized for every Thursday night. At one time, the criterion for earning these parties was a group criterion, and then it was changed to an individual criterion. It was recently moved back so that it was a more publicly known criterion for every child, and the privilege of going to the party was focused on considerably more. Group focus around the parties was found to be a very important reinforcer. Off-unit activities for the children included horseback riding, swimming, movies, spectator sports, hockey, and many others. Home visits were a major source of reinforcers. They were used both to motivate the child to want to go home and to motivate the child to behave while he was on the cottage in order to be allowed to go home.

The program of reinforcers developed with the idea of making the reinforcers not only rewarding but also as therapeutic as possible. It is easy to explain this in relation to food as a reinforcer. Two types of meals, the basic meal and the special meal, were available. The basic meal consisted of a single serving of each of the basic foods, meat and vegetables, and it was served to the child at a table by himself, when he was not able to interact with other children. This meal was always free without earning any marks. The other kind of meal was called a special meal, and the child earned the privilege of having this meal. He received an appetizer and dessert, was served family style, and sat with the other children and staff at a group table. Since it was desirable for the child to sit at the table with the staff and other children, this privilege was a part of the treatment program. The staff wanted him to participate with them in this activity; at the same time, he earned the privilege of doing so. Thus, the relation between the treatment target and the reinforcement was quite explicit. If the child had to pay for the privilege of being there, the probability of his behavior being appropriate at the table with the other children and staff increased. It was rarely necessary to ask a child to leave the dining room when he was at the group table. He was much more inclined to behave appropriately, since he had earned this and had spent his earnings for this kind of privilege. Over a period of time, appropriate social behavior became a part of his habitual repertoire.

Planning for both immediate and long-term reinforcers was an important aspect of the program of reinforcement. In certain situations where there was a need to gain control of the children quickly, an immediate reinforcer was helpful. For example, it was possible to increase the probability of desirable behavior for the entire group in structured activities when it was followed by snacks that were contingent on participation. Immediate reinforcers were good starters for altering behavior quickly in a given situation. These were more important for some children than others and seemed particularly useful for younger children.

On the other hand, if a large number of desirable behaviors were required over a period of time for a home visit, each child who was working to earn the delayed reward was apt to emit a more constant flow of desirable behaviors. It seemed important, over a period of time, to increase long-term or delayed reinforcers.

A balanced budget was important to the program of reinforcers. It was important to budget each child's mark acquisition with potent and frequent reinforcers in order to prevent his building up a large supply of marks and riding on his merits for some time. Although the earning power, cost, and availability of potent reinforcers had to be balanced for each child, at the same time they had to fit into the overall program of available resources, including staff time. Creative use of volunteers was helpful; however, it was important to have regular staff present at all times, to see that the children's programs were being carried out.

Early in the project, an attempt was made to use the data on the number of tokens or marks as a data source. It soon became apparent that this was not a reliable source of information regarding a child's progress. When a behavior that was to be changed for a child was first focused upon, there existed a tendency to reinforce more often, and approximations to the desired behavior were purposefully reinforced more often. In time, as the child reached the terminal behavior and did so more often, the staff seemed to reinforce more intermittently. This manner of staff performance seemed very desirable in terms of maintaining the appropriate behavior for the child. The obvious result, in practice, was that the number of reinforcers decreased in some proportionate way to the increase in desired behavior. With the large number of staff who interacted with a child in a twenty-four-hour period, the proportion of reinforcers, in relation to the rate of emission of desirable behavior at different times during the day, continued to change. Thus, it was not feasible to use the number of reinforcers as an indication of the increase in desired behavior.

At the same time that reinforcing a desirable behavior for one child increased the same desirable behavior in another child, it also could serve to increase an undesirable behavior for a child with different abilities, age, sex, and so forth. The feedback to the child consistently had to indicate appropriate behavior and the fact that the desired item would be available in relation to his emitting appropriate behavior. In addition, the observation of another child who received a particular reinforcer could increase the desirability of that reinforcer. This made it important to use, as much as possible, a range of reinforcers that were appropriate for the entire group of children. When dealing with any exception, the expense of the staff's time was also evaluated.

The Premack principle was used extensively in the program. This principle may be stated as follows: For any pair of activities, the most probable one will reinforce the less probable one. Thus, if the opportunity to engage in the more rewarding activity was made conditional upon the prior performance of low probability activities, then the low probability response increased in frequency. This principle was used with respect to time of activities in the milieu. Low probability activities were scheduled prior to meals, for example, but not prior to leaving for school in the morning. It would be difficult to overemphasize the importance of this principle for group planning; of course, its importance for individual planning should not be minimized.

The relation between the system of feedback and reinforcement (Dimension 4) and the other dimensions is worth noting. This fourth dimension was directed by the three prior dimensions —the plan for progressive movement back into the community (Dimension 1), the development of routine self-care skills (Dimension 2), and the development of appropriate social skills (Dimension 3). The development of appropriate academic skills was also incorporated into the program for each child, and academic performance was reinforced for each child as indicated.

As stated earlier, reinforcers were idiosyncratic. Yet many reinforcers had group meaning or were meaningful or valued by certain social classes or subgroups. The movement scale (Dimension 1) allowed for the opportunity to observe the meaning to the child of a large number of items that might be used as reinforcers. Thus, there was some opportunity to evaluate the incentives or motivations of the child upon entrance into the program at least with respect to the items that were available in the program. The child who was admitted to the program, however, came with many items that had been reinforcing to him in the community and that should not be reinforcing in the milieu.

It became important to alter the meaning of some reinforcers and to substitute other reinforcers. This was a crucial aspect of the treatment procedure and, perhaps, the most difficult. For example, many children who entered the program had been highly reinforced in their undesirable behavior by making adults angry. While it was possible to stop this kind of behavior on the part of the adults who worked with the child in the project, it would continue to be an available potential reinforcer upon returning to the community. Unless the meaning of this adult behavior was changed, the improved behavior would have far less probability of continuing upon discharge. Using this example, it is possible to argue that it is the meaning to the child that should be changed rather than the behavior of the community, i.e. it does not seem wise to encourage the community not to continue to be angry about undesirable behavior. Why should undesirable behavior be ignored by teachers, friends, and parents? The steps and stages in changing the incentive or motivational systems of individuals has been a long-time challenge. The staff attempted to use the system of feedback and reinforcement to increase their skills to change motivation.

The development of the punishment dimension (Dimension 5) is an explicit example of the efforts that were made to conceptualize the project clearly and to develop ways of measuring the results of intervention by the staff.

From the very beginning, a group of grossly undesirable behaviors were labeled and defined for the staff, in order to enable them to act consistently with respect to these behaviors. These behaviors were those that were considered to be sufficiently disruptive, or destructive enough in nature, to jeopardize seriously the effectiveness of the therapeutic program. These were behaviors that could have resulted in injury to the children or personnel, in destruction of property, and in general disruption of the ongoing program. These behaviors generally were classified as assault on the staff or another child, self-destructive behaviors, destruction of property, theft, unauthorized departure from grounds, and sexual deviancy.

In the beginning, other than the categories of behaviors that could be listed as destructive enough to warrant action on the part of the staff, there was no method of classifying deviation. It was necessary to develop the other aspects of the punishment system in relation to the judgment of the staff and to the conditions that existed within the milieu. It was recognized that defiance was a major category of undesirable behavior. To define the behaviors that the staff should ask the children to stop engaging in, or to encourage them, was a difficult task. Also, it was necessary to specify how requests made by staff should be stated in order to be able to know what reaction would constitute a punishable behavior. How to state a request in an explicit, consistent manner was a skill that had to be developed by the staff.

The staff developed the list of undesirable behaviors by rating each behavior that warranted some action on their part in order to stop the behavior and the consequences that they administered. These records were kept for approximately eight months and were used later to develop the present punishment system. From the records kept by the staff, it was possible to compile a comprehensive list of undesirable behaviors that occurred in the milieu. Once the list was compiled, child-care staff and teaching personnel in the Adler school were asked to rank these behaviors according to severity. When the list of undesirable behaviors was ranked according to severity, it was possible to specify the contingencies that the staff should apply to each behavior.

While this chapter has described the milieu, the author does not mean to imply that the treatment conditions were built without consideration for the child. The milieu was built with an awareness of the child and some perceptions of his nature. Chapter 3 is a discussion of the child in the treatment process.

Chapter 3

THE CHILD AND THE TREATMENT PROCESS

A BASIC PREMISE IN THE research project was that people are learners and are able to change. Learning occurs as people interact with their environment over a period of time. Assimilation involves the individual's use of his environment as he conceives it. Experiences are taken in only as far as the individual himself preserves them in terms of his own subjective experience. Thus, the individual experiences an event as he conceives it.

For each child who was admitted to the unit, the following were recognized.

1. The child had experienced a certain amount of the world prior to his admission.

2. The child had assimilated his previous environment in such a way as to have certain expectations, likes, dislikes, attitudes, behaviors, and so forth.

3. The child had developed expectations and ways of coping with the previous environment that were not adequate because of the manner in which he had experienced the previous environment.

4. The child's inadequate ways of coping, when they consisted of unacceptable behavior, would have a tendency, if ignored, to be reinforced or rewarded by the attentions of other children in the milieu.

5. The child would have to be encouraged to adapt to major aspects of the milieu through setting up a flow of influences in the immediate situation that were strong enough to exert a pull on the child to act according to the requirements of the situation.

6. The child would have to understand what would be required of him in the milieu, in order for him to be an active participant in his own treatment process.

It is important to state that there was respect for the individual child. Opportunities were offered for him to develop the strengths that he possessed and to increase his repertoire of acceptable behaviors and skills. A child's total history, his attitudes, or his feelings—with respect to setting up his treatment programs—were not taken into account, however, at all times. In the approach that was used to deal with or to treat the individual child, it was impossible to consider the whole individual at all times. The strengths or weaknesses of the child, which were relevant to each situation, were given consideration at each point in time.

The established environment needed to have such an impact on the child that the child would conceive and incorporate the environmental experience as it had been structured and would find it difficult to miss the deliberate cues. Requirements were conveyed to the child both verbally and behaviorally. Verbal and nonverbal communication were vital to the process, e.g. the child was told what was required of him; he saw other children rewarded for doing the required; and he saw the staff model the required behaviors in the established environment.

In addition to establishing respect for the child, the milieu was set up in such a way as to teach the child to respect other people. In this way, people became meaningful to him.

Appropriate ways of handling anger or frustration were taught to the child. With some children, attention was called to appropriate ways simply by letting the child tell the staff the alternative ways that he could have handled the situation. A child was encouraged to do this by rewarding him for telling how he could have handled it more appropriately. Later he was rewarded for handling the situation more appropriately.

For the child who was unable to verbalize or even think about a more appropriate or alternative way of handling anger or frustration, an attempt was made to set up opportunities for the child to witness alternative ways, or ways were suggested verbally and/or demonstrated. This was accomplished by pointing out the appropriate behaviors of other people or in miniature role-playing situations. At times, it was necessary to start simply by making the child aware of the inappropriateness of his behavior in the situation and later by making him aware of alternative appropriate ways.

It was important that the child's coping patterns, i.e. the characteristic way that he was observed to interact with or behave toward the flow of influences, were assessed accurately enough so that requirements beyond his reach were not established. Attention was also given to the child's coping capacity, i.e. the characteristic strength and weakness of the child that had been inferred on the basis of his observed coping patterns.

Programs were set up for the child that enabled him to progress toward a desired terminal pattern of behavior (Dimension 1). The programs communicated to the child what was required of him (Dimensions 2 and 3); how he was able to receive positive attention from the staff, rewards, and privileges (Dimension 4); and how to discriminate between desirable and undesirable behavior (Dimension 5).

In the Orientation Level (Dimension 1) of the program, it was possible to tell from the child's verbal and nonverbal behavior that certain activities, things, and people were more important to him than others. Behavior was recognized at the child's level of meaning, i.e. each child placed different interpretations and values on objects, behavior, people, and so forth. These observed preferences were used to set up the child's reinforcement or reward program (Dimension 4), which was used to motivate him to behave appropriately in order to earn a meaningful reward.

On the other hand, care was taken not to interpret or infer particular meaning of the child's behavior in setting up the treatment programs for him, i.e. inferences or interpretation of behavior rarely were made. Staff did not infer that certain objects in the established environment should represent certain things to the child; instead the programs were set up in such a way that they taught meanings and values to the child.

Prosocial behaviors (Dimensions 2 and 3 plus academic skills) were involved principally in the child's treatment program. The problems or the behavior that had been the cause of the child's admission to the unit were discussed openly with him, but they were not a focal point in his treatment program in the same way that the prosocial behaviors were. It was not assumed that the child needed to rid himself of negative attitudes toward people, either verbally or behaviorally. Instead of dealing with his past experiences and helping him to verbalize these or to act out pent-up feelings, he was taught to deal with frustration and anger as it occurred in a given situation. For example, if something happened to him in the milieu that angered him and he reacted to this anger by hitting another child, then he was punished.

The content or curriculum of the program offered opportunities for participation, interaction, sharing, helping, cooperation, and independent constructive behavior (Dimension 3). It was important in the program to keep the child occupied constructively. If the child was involved actively in prosocial behaviors, he was not involved actively in antisocial behaviors. It was more important that the child spent his time doing appropriate things than that he spent his time being punished for inappropriate behavior.

The child was made aware that he would be punished consistently for inappropriate behavior as it occurred. The process that was set up for teaching the child to discriminate between desirable and undesirable behavior was twofold. At the same time that the process communicated that a behavior was unacceptable, an attempt was made to communicate that appropriate behavior was not only acceptable but also was rewarded and was satisfying to the staff. Instead of ignoring undesirable behavior, it was dealt with according to the punishment system (Dimension 5). The action taken communicated to the child, in a very explicit way, that the behavior was inappropriate. The system said very clearly that you do not hit people, but you do help other people.

In the treatment program, the notion of adaptation was separated from the notion of creativity. Although the program was set up to help the child adapt or conform to the expectation of the milieu, it was not intended to stifle creativity. Activities of the milieu needed to offer opportunities for appropriate creativity; therefore, arts and crafts, dramatics, dancing, leadership roles, games, and so forth, were a major part of the content of the milieu.

The treatment program for a child was altered if it did not

influence his behavior positively. His program was altered (a) when the quality of the child's coping patterns was such that he failed consistently to utilize the opportunities that were presented to him; (b) when the quality of the child's coping pattern was such that he continued to be disruptive to the milieu; or (c) when the child's coping patterns in the environment altered the environment, i.e. if his flow of influence in the environment was such that it was destructive to the environment or increased inappropriate behavior in the environment.

Assessment was made of what changes were required for the coping process to develop in a positive manner for all those involved. It seems important, however, to point out again that this kind of assessment was made by looking at the flow of influences. A review was made of the requirements, of the feedback and reinforcement system, and of the child's pattern of undesirable behavior in the punishment system. The measurement or the evaluation of the programs was such that if the flow of influences increased the probability of desirable human actions, then the objectives had been reached. If it decreased the probability of these human actions, then the objectives had not been reached.

The framework of the dimensions served as guidelines which aided the child to understand that it would be possible for him to attain his own goals. Each participated daily in the collection of information relevant to his individual treatment program. Development of the instruments used by the staff in assembling a record of each child's decrease or increase of desirable behavior are presented in Chapter 4.

Chapter 4

INSTRUMENTS FOR RESEARCH - PROJECT EVALUATION

In designing the research project, an effort was made to build into it a matrix of interlocking measures by which it could be evaluated. Since most projects cannot afford to have a large research staff, but should not be excused from the obligation of evaluation, one of the goals was to try to use, as much as possible, the direct-care staff in data collection. To be maximally useful, data must be processed as it is collected so that the program may be monitored on a continuing basis. To this end, data were recorded in a form designed for automated data processing on an off-line basis. An ultimate goal for another project of this type could be to have direct-care staff record the data on an on-line basis through the use of a remote terminal in the project office. One of the biggest hurdles of the project was to feed back, in a meaningful fashion, the results of the continuing evaluation to the child-care staff, Adler teachers and Extramural Case Coordinators.

The instruments that were used most extensively in the research project are described in detail in this chapter in the following order.

1. Daily Checklist.
2. Mark Sheet.
3. Special Behavior Report Form.
4. Independent Observations.

Appendix B provides samples of each instrument and also the instructions furnished to the staff for filling out the Special Behavior Report Forms. Data obtained from these instruments was processed on an IBM 360/75 computer at the Digital Computer Laboratory of the University of Illinois.

Daily Checklist

The Daily Checklist was completed by the cottage staff for each child every day that the child was in the cottage. The check list indicated the completion or absence of specific behaviors that were labeled as MAB (Dimension 2). The MAB or minimal appropriate behaviors tapped the more simple of the child's prosocial behaviors. The MABs were concentrated in situations such as getting up, preparing for and consuming meals, getting off to school, and preparing for and going to bed.

The reliability of the Daily Checklist was defined in terms of percent agreement between two people filling out the check list for the same child at the same time. Since the behaviors were easily observed if staff were present, the emphasis in the reliability checks was to see whether staff recorded the behaviors. Reliability checks were made without informing the cottage staff that a second person was filling out a check list. The second person was typically a member of the research-project staff. All staff were familiar with the instrument, and their presence did not arouse suspicion.

Reliability checks on the Daily Checklist were made during July and November, 1969. Table I also provides reliability data for items that were found to be below the overall reliabilities and for items that were added, eliminated, or modified on the Daily Checklist between reliability checks.

How the Data Was Analyzed

The data was subdivided into three groups of (a) tokened items, (b) nontokened items, and (c) Premacked items. This subdivision of the items varied from child to child depending on his program, and they were computer analyzed individually to show the percent performance during each week.

The measure of percent performance of MAB items was one of several indices of appropriate performance. On the Orientation Level (Dimension 1) when behaviors were observed without systematic application of contingencies, the Daily Checklist served as an indicator of the type of MABs already in the child's repertoire. Nonperformance of MABs in the absence of contin-

TABLE I
OVERALL RELIABILITY OF THE DAILY CHECKLIST

Item	July 1969 82.6%	Nov. 1969 83.0%	Item Changes Between July and November	
			Items Added	Items Eliminated
Out of bed on time	66	30		
Makes bed	80	100		
Dressed neatly	80	92		
Hair neat	78	76		
Room neat	80	69		
Wash hands (B)	100			X
On time (B)	100	100		
Quiet going to dining room (B)	100			X
Appropriate table manners (B)	93	92		
Brush teeth (B)	42	75		
Arrives school on time (B)	93	76		
No disturbance en route school	92			X
Wash hands (L)	100	71		
Quiet going to dining room (L)	100			
On time (L)	90	100		
Appropriate table manners (L)	78	80		
Brush teeth (L)	94	100		
Closets and drawers neat	80	53		
Arrives school on time (L)	88	25		
No disturbance en route school	100			X
Wash hands (D)	50	100		
Quiet going to dining room (D)	75			X
On time (D)	100	100		
Appropriate table manners (D)	100	90		
Brush teeth (D)	36	90		
Takes shower	100	90		
Put out laundry	66	90		
In bed on time	73	72		X
Remains in room	66			X
Quiet after retiring	45			X
Appropriate social behavior (B)		92	X	
Appropriate social behavior (L)		80	X	
Appropriate social behavior (D)		81	X	
Dressed appropriately for bed		66	X	

gencies only provided the information that the child was not emitting these behaviors. Performance in the absence of contingencies did say something about the availability of the behaviors. High performance during Orientation Level in the absence of contingencies was more typical than nonperformance. On the treatment levels of Dimension 1, contingencies were applied to MAB items that had a low frequency of occurrence during Orientation Level. Low initial performance that was followed by rapid increase in performance after the application of contingencies also suggested the availability of the behaviors.

Later in a child's program, clusters of MABs were typically linked with Premack contingencies. This was one of the ways that tokening was phased out, and the more natural contingencies were phased into a child's program in preparation for his return to the community.

The types of behaviors recorded on the Daily Checklist changed little over time. Changes were made with respect to the types of consequences that were attached to the performance of the behaviors and to the way in which the data was analyzed.

Originally the items were divided into tokened and nontokened groups. The consequences for performance of a particular item was constant across all children in the program. Later items had token or Premack contingencies applied to them, depending upon the decisions of each child's Intramural Counselor and Extramural Case Coordinator. The breakdown of items into tokened and nontokened groups was intended to provide a measure of differential reinforcement. There was definite problems that were related to the interpretation of this breakdown of data. It was difficult to establish the comparability of items. It was not possible to say that under the method first implemented that the difficulty of the set of nontokened items was equal to that of the tokened items. It was true also that for certain of the untokened items, informal contingencies were developed by cottage staff to insure eventual performance.

Mark Sheet

The Mark Sheet was prepared by cottage staff and was carried daily by each child. The sheet indicated the child's target behaviors for his program, through the grouping and labeling of a series of $\frac{1}{4} \times \frac{1}{2}$ inch boxes, and the number of marks that a child could earn in a day by emitting these target behaviors. Appendix B contains three sample Mark Sheets that demonstrate the colors employed by the staff to differentiate whether the child was on response-cost (yellow) or time-out (white) punishment condition and to identify the sheet used to record school marks (blue).

The cottage staff used inked markers to stamp each staff's number in an appropriate box when the child performed a specified behavior, and they used indelible pens to cross marks off as they were spent by a child. The staff recorded for what the marks were spent on the Mark Sheet. In addition to paying fines on the response-cost punishment condition, the child could spend his marks to purchase something (Dimension 4).

A daily summary of the number of marks earned and for what the child spent his marks was recorded in each child's data book (Chapter 6, "Communication Channels"). The Mark Sheets provided a record of which staff were giving marks and how frequently. These data were analyzed only occasionally to obtain information about the frequency with which each staff issued marks.

The Mark Sheet had daily uses. It was an immediately available reminder to child and staff of the target behaviors for each child's treatment program. The number of marks earned in a particular category was a popular means for the Intramural Counselor and the cottage staff to determine when various criteria for a child's daily or weekly reward had been reached. The sheets provided information about the types of things and activities that a child was buying, i.e. what things were reinforcing for him, and the sheets were a symbolic record of daily achievement that the child could talk about and for which he could receive praise.

The Mark Sheets also provided the Intramural Counselor with some idea of how difficult the child's individual program was for the child and how positive the attitude of the staff in general was toward the child. A child who was earning far below the maximum allowed by his program might be in trouble either or both ways. Staff members were encouraged to give plenty of marks for approximations of desired behavior. They were encouraged to maintain appropriate behavior on a rich schedule of marks and then to decrease gradually the number of marks used to maintain the behavior. This procedure did not allow the number of marks received to be used as a reliable index to the frequency of the child's target behaviors.

Special Behavior Report Form

Every time a cottage staff invoked a punishment contingency, time out or response cost, a Special Behavior Report Form was completed by the cottage staff. After the invoking of the initial contingency, continued punishable behaviors and escalating punishable behavior were recorded on the same sheet. The Special Behavior Report Form contained space for a narrative of the antecedent events, a description of the undesirable behavior, and the consequent events. Baseline data for each child was recorded during his Orientation Level. Examples of the three kinds of Special Behavior Report Forms, i.e. time out, response cost, and baseline, are presented in Appendix B, and instructions furnished to staff for completing these forms are also provided.

How the Data Was Analyzed

The data was computer analyzed on a daily basis and provided a listing of the number of initial contingencies invoked for each category, number of intervals of continued punishable behavior for each category, number of intervals of subsequent punishable behavior for each category, and a summary of the total frequency of all punishable behavior emitted for the day.

The Special Behavior Report Form provided the data used in the punishment study (Chapter 8). Punishment-study graphs, which showed the mean frequency of punishable behavior per three-day blocks, were used extensively as indices of change by the Intramural Counselors. Finer breakdowns of the incidence of punishable behavior by categories were available to the Intramural Counselors in each child's data book.

The narratives of events on the forms detailed information about what punishable behavior occurred and with whom, i.e. staff, peer group, or particular children. The Special Behavior Report Forms were used to ascertain when a child had the most trouble. They provided information about the child's acceptance of punishment contingencies, e.g. how long it took him to quiet down in time out, escalating punishable behavior, and continuing punishable behavior. It also provided information about the distribution of the invoking of contingencies across cottage staff. With the implementation of a pilot punishment study and the punishment study (Chapter 8), the instrument developed greatly with respect to the range of behaviors it recorded and the degree of specification of behavior it provided. From December, 1968, to April, 1969, the instrument also provided data on the child's response to an interview that was conducted by cottage staff in order to help the child establish cognitively the relation of his behavior to the punishment.

Independent Observations

One of the principle dependent variables consisted of time samples of the children's behavior that were recorded by non-cottage staff who were hired on an hourly basis to observe the children, to record their observations using the categories of the instrument, and to compile and summarize the data they gathered. They were trained and supervised by the research assistants. They were typically students at the University of Illinois and remained with the research project for about a year on the average. The observers were not allowed to interact with the children or staff. Similarly the children and staff were instructed not to engage the observers in any interaction.

Observations were made Monday through Friday from 9:00 to 11:00 A.M. and 1:00 to 2:30 P.M. in the Adler School and from 6:00 to 9:00 P.M. on the cottage. Observations also were made Saturday morning on the cottage from 8:00 A.M. to 12:00 noon. At times, budgetary restrictions forced the implementation of more abbreviated schedules of observation.

Initially, the observers rated individual children for a block of time up to 20 minutes. The procedure was changed so that the observers rotated their observations after two minutes and moved from one child to the next on a prescribed random schedule. In the summer of 1969, an attempt was made to observe the child again for a block of time but only in a particular situation, such as gym period or study hall. Sampling behavior on a predetermined random schedule for short intervals of time seemed to produce less variable data than sampling large chunks of behavior on an unspecified schedule. There was still question as to whether the sampling of broader time spans of behavior in the same situation produced more variable data than the random sampling of two-minute blocks of behavior.

The observational instrument was set up to provide a framework for the target behaviors that focused on types of interaction (objects, self, peer, staff, group) and on quality of interactions (deviant or nondeviant). In addition, the behavior was classified as verbal or motor action (Appendix B, "Independent Observations Handbook"). It was intended that specific target categories would be plugged in and out of the more general framework. The systematic addition and subtraction of target behaviors, however, was dependent on a clearer conceptualization of task related to prosocial behaviors (Dimension 3). Consequently, this dependent variable measure remained a global measure of interactions. Because types of deviant behavior were less frequent than types of appropriate behavior, the strategy was to identify and set criteria for behavior that was deviant and to classify, by elimination, all other behaviors as appropriate.

The following is a schematic representation of the classifications:

Positive Staff Reaction	Negative Staff Reaction	Neutral Staff Reaction

	Objects	Self	Peer	Staff	Group
Verbal					
Fine Motor					
Gross Motor					
Inactive					

Any observed behavior was placed into one of these categories. For example, if the child was alone in the activity room talking, the behavior was rated Verbal-Self-Deviant. Appendix B contains additional examples of how the behaviors fitted into the observational classifications.

When behavior occurred that was not previously defined as deviant but which cottage staff and/or observers felt might be added to the compendium of deviant behavior, the behavior was discussed, and some decision about its inclusion and criteria was made by the research staff. No behavior was rated deviant until it was officially defined and included in the Independent Observations Handbook.

Observations were made while the children were in class, having free periods from class, and on the cottage. Situations in the classroom included independent seat work, group games with the teacher, group discussions, and semistructured periods, when art and science projects were done. Since there were a large number of different types of situations that could occur in the classroom, the classification of behavior as deviant or nondeviant varied intentionally to fit the different situations. For example, when the class was doing independent seat work, talking out without first being recognized was not rated deviant. Reliability in such a system depended very much upon well-defined structuring of the different situations so that the observers were clear as to what criteria they were to use. On the cottage, the situations observed typically included meals, snacks, structured and unstructured group activities, study hall, outdoor free play, and off-unit activities, such as bowling, swimming, pool, and shopping trips.

The reliability for this instrument was conceptualized in terms of the proportion of observations made that were in agreement out of the total number of observations that were possible. In order for the ratings of two observers to be in agreement, they had to be identical with respect to the topographical category, the interaction category, and the evaluative category, i.e. deviant or nondeviant. In addition, when both observers left the same boxes blank on the Observer's Rating Sheet to indicate the nonoccurrence of those behaviors, this was also counted as an agreement. Appendix B contains an example of the Observer's Rating Sheet and also of the Observer's Summary Sheet, which was prepared by the independent observers for the IBM key puncher.

The reliability data is presented in Table II. The percent agreement across all children was close to 90 for both the cottage and the Adler school.

TABLE II
RELIABILITY DATA FOR INDEPENDENT OBSERVATIONS

Subject Number	Cottage		School	
	Average Reliability	Av. No. Days between Rel. Checks	Average Reliability	Av. No. Days between Rel. Checks
1	79.4	5	—	—
2	83.4	4	85.9	10
3	83.8	5	92.3	5
4	87.3	4	90.6	22
5	85.5	5	83.1	5
6	82.1	5	92.2	9
7	91.0	8	91.5	8
8	86.9	4	85.7	6
9	89.0	11	86.8	14
10	91.7	7	93.5	13
11	92.1	9	88.3	11
12	92.8	6	88.3	6
13	89.2	9	86.9	8
14	91.1	9	90.8	9
15	89.0	11	92.0	8
16	91.5	12	93.0	14
17	89.4	9	89.4	12
18	89.3	9	89.7	13
19	91.2	16	91.8	7
20	90.3	12	93.8	10
21	86.9	14	87.0	28
22	89.0	10	87.4	22
23	88.2	11	95.0	20
24	89.2	23	89.5	31
25	92.8	33	—	—
26	90.3	6	100.0	1
27	87.7	23	96.2	12
28	83.3	13	89.4	21
29	—	—	92.0	11
30	—	—	—	—

The independent observations made up a large bulk of the data used by the research staff to evaluate progress. Graphs of the percent deviant measure and other categories, especially peer, staff, and group interactions, were commonly used by the Adler and the research staff in their periodic reviews of a child's progress.

Other Instruments

Previous discussion has been limited to those instruments in use at the termination of the research project. The following is a brief discussion of the instruments that were supplanted or discarded in the development of the project.

Token Earning

Until the revision of the method of feedback and the distribution of reinforcers (Dimension 4), token earning was used as a major index of progress. The number of plastic tokens that were earned in school and on the cottage, for the performance of minimal appropriate behaviors and of appropriate social behaviors, was recorded and played an important part in determining when a child advanced in his program and when he had reached the criteria for special contingencies.

The progressive revisions in the project emphasized communication of the target behaviors and a more natural process of removing the tokens as the behavior became a regular part of the child's activity. Thus, the plastic tokens were replaced by the Mark Sheet. It was recognized that token earning was not an index of desirable change, and this type of data ceased to be used as an index of progress.

Behavior Description Form

The Behavior Description Form provided an organized way for staff to describe appropriate or inappropriate behavior that they felt was particularly noteworthy. The form provided for proper identification of date, child, and so forth and for a description of the antecedents to the behavior, the behavior, and the consequences of the behavior. The information obtained on this form was used to develop the punishment study (Chapter 8). The Behavior Description Form was discontinued when the Special Behavior Report Form was developed.

Rating Checklist

In the early months of the project, one cottage worker was assigned to rate one child at the end of a shift on the Rating Checklist. The Rating Checklist consisted of the six categories of appropriate social behaviors (Dimension 3) and categories of inappropriate behaviors, such as assault, defiance, and verbal abuse. Reliability was taken weekly, i.e. once a week two workers rated the same child independently. The amount of agreement between ratings was low. Since the two workers doing the ratings rarely had equal exposure to the child, global ratings for the entire day could not always be expected to agree. Under such conditions, where estimates of reliability were obtained from unequal samples of behavior, it was decided that it was not possible to determine reliability. This instrument was discarded in the summer of 1968.

Chapter 5

CHILD-CARE TRAINING FOR RESEARCH-PROJECT STAFF

TRAINING for the research-project staff was continuous throughout the project. In the initial stage of the project, there were fourteen days of training for the entire staff. These two weeks were more formal sessions, and the teaching methods used were lecture, role playing, discussion, and written exercises. Since there was a constant turnover of staff, and one or two members were added at a time, the training became more that of learning from other staff members, plus small training groups for short periods of time. Time was arranged, however, for a day each month to be used for training. These sessions were less formal than the original training sessions. The staff was much more active in the training process and the material used for discussion was taken from experience on the unit.

All training, whether given in the initial period, monthly sessions, individual supervision, or modeled by other staff, contained the orientation and content as presented in the following discussion.

The training program emphasized the fact that children never come alone. Areas considered in the training program were those related to the child, i.e. the Adler Zone Center, the individual child's family, other agencies including foster homes, and the Children's Research Center.

The research-project staff was introduced to the Adler Zone Center's organization and philosophy of continuity of care. Particular attention was given to the role of the Extramural Case Coordinator since he was the person who would know the child first and would be responsible for his return to the community. The mutual dependency of the Extramural Case Coordinator and the Intramural Counselor was discussed, the role of the child's teacher was explained, and emphasis was placed on the need for constant communication between these people. The staff also was introduced to the dietary, plant maintenance, and housekeeping staffs; the interdependency that exists in the functions of those involved in the child's care and treatment again was emphasized.

The second area of the training program, the individual child's family, recognized that the family had been a part of the child's life for a long time. It was pointed out that the family carried the responsibility for the child longer than anyone in the agency and that the family consisted of the people who were not only those most involved in the child's life but also those most important with respect to his total treatment program. The tendency to blame parents for the child's behavior was discussed, emphasizing the need to consider constructive approaches to helping the parent cope with his child's behavior.

The role that other agencies had played and/or would play in the lives of many children was considered. It was pointed out that some of the children who came to the project had been placed in other institutions and foster homes previously; some would return to institutions or foster homes; and some would enter other state-care situations upon leaving Adler. Since other resources for children were administered by a variety of other agencies, the need for planning and working with these resources was vital to the care of the children.

The organization and purpose of the Children's Research Center was explained to the staff. Many discussions focused around the relation of research to clinical practice. The research-project staff was taught that research is the evaluation of clinical practice, but that the thinking of a researcher and a clinical practitioner should not be different. Each should be interested in what it is that is being done that contributes to the child's treatment. If the researcher and practitioner are able to state together the interventive act (independent variable) and the criterion for desired change (dependent variable), then both are involved in a search for answers to practice questions. Each has a vested interest in the knowledge to be obtained, and data collection becomes a vital part of the treatment process. It was further pointed out that change often occurs more slowly in research projects since research procedures require time to collect and analyze data; that this is not always necessary in practice; and that practice, however, has made many swings as a result of not adequately evaluating the data.

The material was presented through brief descriptions of situations, discussion sessions, and role-playing exercises. The role-playing exercises consisted of members of the Adler staff talking to other agency people about plans for a child and of Extramural Case Coordinators discussing a child with a member of another agency or a parent. There were sessions in which the child-care trainees discussed the coordination between services and suggested ways that coordination could be implemented better.

The training program was structured further around the following areas:

1. Dimensions of the milieu.
2. Cottage management.
3. Recreation and arts and crafts activities.
4. School and cottage coordination.
5. Physical health and drugs.
6. Observation and recording.
7. Individual child care.

The concept of continuity of care was basic to the training program, i.e. the idea that the process of bringing the child in, treating him and sending him back into the community should have a continuity that would enable the child to obtain maximum profit from the experience of having been in residence at the research-project cottage.

Dimensions of the Milieu

In training the staff around the dimensions, it was emphasized that these dimensions were established in an attempt to develop a milieu and to serve as guidelines for the research project. It was important that the child-care staff understood how the dimensions fitted into the operation. A part of the research was to see how readily the staff could adapt, did adapt, or did not adapt to the dimensions.

Child-Care Training for Research-Project Staff   53

The content and use of these dimensions was discussed in Chapter 2. In addition to presenting the content, certain attitudes and skills were emphasized as we taught each of these dimensions.

The research cottage had a system of progression from admission to discharge (Dimension 1). An important notion that was emphasized in the teaching of Dimension 1 was the importance of planning for the child to return to the community, i.e. to rehabilitate him so that he could function in the community. Also emphasized was the fact that action needed to be taken many times with respect to the community, as well as the child, during his stay on the unit.

In teaching the system of progression back into the community, it was important to recognize with the staff how other agencies and other services were necessary to bring the child back into the community. It was very important to emphasize with the child-care staff that regularly the community does not get ready for the child to return; and it works two ways in that the child also has to make some alterations to return to the community. It was very easy for the people who worked directly with the child to become very blaming with respect to other people, particularly parents, and very impatient because other people did not furnish what staff felt to be necessary requirements for the child to return to the community. The staff often identified so much with the child that they were unable to see the problems that he created for other people. It was necessary to continue to help the staff to understand the complexities of the community and to understand that although the unit was set up to help the child get back into the community, it was still to some extent an artificial community and was possible to control many things that are not controlled in the outside world. That it was important to get the child ready for this, as well as to get the community ready for the return of the child, was emphasized.

In teaching the system of progression, the Premack principle was a major concept that was taught. Usually children were started with quite concrete reinforcement and moved to a system that was much more feasible and in keeping with the setting to which they would return. This was taught with the use of the

Premack principle. The idea was to help the child to sustain the desirable behaviors with the reinforcers that existed in the community. Attention was also given to building-in successful experiences for the children and to allowing them ample opportunity to feel pride in their own success so that this could continue to be a very strong reinforcer and motivater in the community. The staff was taught to express considerable excitement with respect to returning to the public schools, to going home, and to being able to stay home.

In the beginning, much of the training around the daily routine and the minimum acceptable behaviors (Dimension 2) was accomplished through lectures because the staff was not experienced in trying to get a child to brush his teeth or to get out of bed. Role playing was used to show how this was done. Particular attention was given to awarding tokens or marks for a child's accomplishments. Much time was spent in relating award giving to the total structure of the cottage. Attention was given also to the need for a daily routine time to accomplish the tasks that were listed in the MABs and to record them.

The categories of the socially acceptable behaviors (Dimension 3) were taught to the staff. Experience demonstrated that teaching categories was a difficult task. As pointed out in Chapter 2, it was found that the staff concretized the categories and each category became more a discrete behavior than a category of behaviors into which you could fit many individual patterns of behavior.

It is the author's opinion that this occurred because there was not the awareness of teaching categories that there was of teaching the discrete behaviors. Instead, it would have been possible to teach the staff the many ways that a child could behave within a category at different levels of skill. In addition, there was some confusion over the fact that these categories were being used as guidelines for desirable behavior at the same time that they were being used for tallying the behavior. Thus, staff were much more concerned about keeping up with whether or not the child interacted, and the need for giving tokens at that time, than with thinking of the variety of ways that this could be used for individual programming. It took a very long time to separate these ideas in the minds of the staff members. The difference between abstract thinking, concrete observable behaviors, and guidelines for individual treatment programs needed to be made clear in the training program.

The feedback and reinforcement system (Dimension 4) was explained. The importance of communicating to the child what was expected of him and when he had accomplished an expected behavior was the major emphasis in this dimension.

Rate and time was important in the giving of reinforcers. It was understood that in treatment programs and in natural settings almost all reinforcers are given intermittently. There seemed to be a "natrual" progressive decrease in reinforcing target behaviors. The staff tended to give more marks in the beginning and then to weed out slowly as the behavior began to increase so that rate, with respect to giving reinforcers, seemed to take care of itself. It did not seem to be something that needed to be taught so specifically. However, calling attention to the immediacy of reinforcement was important. To teach the use of successive approximations was necessary. The staff as a whole tended to look for terminal behavior and to reinforce terminal behavior unless they were specifically taught to do otherwise.

In teaching the reinforcement system, particular emphasis was given to pairing social reinforcers with any concrete reinforcers. Discussion of hoarding things and whether or not to allow layaway, charge plans, buying on time, etc., were important in teaching staff to use a program of reinforcers.

In training the staff to use a punishment system (Dimension 5), the staff was taught the importance of setting up rules, of establishing categories of punishable behavior, and of timing the punishment.

The staff was taught not to set up situations that encouraged the child to be defiant. Staff was taught to think about the reasonableness of a demand, and that it was better to suggest a desirable alternative behavior than to immediately punish an undesirable behavior. This skill was not readily taught by lecture; however, by emphasizing its importance and with experience, the staff members gained in their skill of diverting the undesirable behavior into more appropriate channels.

The staff was taught not to ignore undesirable behavior. They were taught to divert the process that was leading to an undesirable behavior into a process leading to a desirable behavior. They were also taught that if a unit rule was broken, then the specific contingency was applied. The staff was taught to say verbally or nonverbally, "That is a behavior that is not tolerated in this unit," or in other words, "We just do not do that here."

Cottage Management

The importance of cottage management was discussed in the training program. The importance of communications, the need to plan for time to communicate between shifts, the means of communicating information at shift time, and scheduling daily activities were noted. During this part of the training program, the structure of the milieu administration was explained to the staff.

Communication was a major emphasis in all aspects of the training program, but the importance of establishing a time and place for communication was the emphasis in the cottage management aspects of the training. The staff was taught to read all bulletin boards and other materials or records at the beginning of each shift. They were taught where and how to record relevant events at the end of each shift.

Scheduling regular appointments with teachers, Extramural Case Coordinators, and other involved personnel was emphasized. In addition, the importance of setting aside time to communicate with individual children was taught. Also, the staff was taught the importance of establishing a time when the children could talk with representative members of the staff about group concerns.

The author noted that many schemes were established for communication of different aspects of the program. At different stages of the program, different means were used. They were taught, however, that as much as possible information should be communicated in written form.

The entire staff needed to know the schedule of daily activities, and each staff member was taught to assume responsibility for whatever area was assigned to him. Additional training was given the shift leader to enable them to coordinate the staff and activities.

The staff members were taught to anticipate the amount of time that would be required for each aspect of the activities, and they were given exercises in planning the day's activities, beginning with getting the children up in the morning and ending with getting the children to bed at night. Discussion was led around the children's school programs and the number of child-care workers who would be required to relieve the school situation. As soon as all activities became a routine part of the child-care worker's functioning, he was able to turn his attention to the individual child.

Recreation and Arts and Crafts Activities

When outlining the daily activities, certain amounts of time were scheduled for recreation and arts and crafts. Different ways of using the time scheduled were discussed, as were the kinds of activities that could be used for the children as a group and for individual children to enhance their total program.

Since the child-care workers often were not familiar with games and activities that were popular with children at this age, it was necessary to teach the staff the games and activities and to train the staff to teach the children. Role playing was conducted around such things as beginning game activities with the children, how to anticipate activities so that the children would be interested in an event when it occurred, and how to deal with inappropriate behavior in the activity situation.

The staff was involved in discussions about group activities and the individual child. They were taught to tolerate exceptions to group participation and not to invoke a defiance contingency as long as the child was not misbehaving in addition to not participating. This was an opportunity to teach shaping and the idea of successive approximation to the staff. It was explained that group enthusiasm about an activity made the activity more reinforcing for the children and was more likely to involve each child. Staff members were taught that to get the child to talk about a game, once it was over, would increase the possibility of his participating the next time. Prior to this, however, the game had to be allowed to develop without confronting the child about nonparticipation.

School and Cottage Coordination

Since school activities were a large part of the child's day, the techniques and problems in coordinating school and cottage activities were presented to the staff. Attention was given to the teacher's expectations with respect to homework, and the role that Intramural Counselors were to assume. Other areas covered were (a) how to handle the child who refused to go to school; (b) the part that the child-care worker played in getting the child to school and into the classroom; and (c) what measures to take when the child had to be removed from the school and returned to the cottage.

The relationship between the teacher's role and the child-care worker's role was delineated clearly for the teacher and staff. It was not so important how these roles were handled as it was that each understood his role. Role-playing sessions were used to teach this. The staff evaluated the sessions and discussed the problems involved in communication between child-care worker and teacher, in consistency with respect to discipline, and in developing appropriate school attitudes. The staff member who accompanied the children to school had to model appropriate behaviors, e.g. going from cottage to school, entering the halls, and greeting the teachers.

Most of the children who came into the research project had experienced school previously and knew that school was for academic activities that differed from the cottage activities. The staff was trained to relate differently to the school atmosphere than to the cottage atmosphere.

Physical Health and Drugs

The relationship between the child-care staff and the nursing and medical staff was discussed. Common pediatric illnesses were presented to the staff, and basic indicators of physical illness were discussed. Methods of determining when a child was ill and the procedure to follow when a child was injured or ill were taught to the staff.

An exercise in which the trainee related to the problem of physical illness was given in the training session. The trainee followed through the procedure outlined to be used in case of a child's illness. There also was an exercise in ways of administering drugs to a child. Role-playing sessions involved methods of dealing with a child who was suspected of malingering or who had problems that were psychosomatic. These were dealt with, discussed, and evaluated by the staff.

Observation and Recording

Observation and recording were handled in the training program through lecture and discussion. Reliability factors and the distinction between facts and inferences were emphasized. The three-term contingency (ABC) was introduced as a recording framework, i.e. the antecedent behavior, the behavior, and the consequences of the behavior. For undesirable behavior, the staff was taught to record the antecedent behavior, the undesirable behavior, and the consequences that were invoked.

Means and methods of collecting and displaying data were discussed, with particular emphasis on the use of graphs. Each trainee was asked to write an incident report. These reports were read to the group and were discussed and criticized by the group.

All forms (Chapter 4) that were used by cottage staff were introduced. Staff members were asked to use these forms to record behaviors demonstrated by other staff members in role-playing sessions. The staff needed to know all forms very well in order to use them competently without giving them undue attention. Experience showed that the more useful the form, the more apt the staff member was to record the data. Constant monitoring of data recording by staff was necessary because staff tended to become lax in spite of the attention given to this in the training sessions. It was found that when staff received feedback about the research, they were more attentive to recording on the forms.

Since individual staff members interpreted what happened in a given incident quite differently, their own behavior was available to train them to be careful of inferences that they made about specific behavior. If this was done too soon in the training program, however, the amount of anxiety exhibited by the trainees was extreme, and they found it difficult to tolerate this aspect of the training.

Individual Child Care

Each trainee was asked to prepare a daily schedule for a child that included the specific targets for the individual child's program and the activities that required his participation as a member of the group. These schedules were prepared in detail with brief descriptions of each of the activities, and they were discussed, criticized, and evaluated by the entire staff.

It was difficult to teach the staff to develop a program for an individual child prior to the staff's having experienced a similar kind of problem. The trainees used textbook examples for very discrete problems, such as toilet training or speech development. It proved more profitable to help the trainees themselves to model a behavior for each other, to use it, to relate to the child's lack of skill, and then to plan a program for developing the skill in relation to the child's own idiosyncratic way of behaving. Prior to working with the individual child, the training program allowed the trainees the opportunity to shape each other's behavior and to use themselves as reinforcers. In so doing, they participated in exercises that were designed to show another affection, praise, and adverse reactions; and this made them conscious of the use of themselves in the treatment process. After these sessions, the group participated in evaluating how well the staff member who was playing the role communicated his pleasure or displeasure. In addition, the staff members who observed the role playing were asked to record the number of times that reinforcement was displayed and that displeasure was shown in order to help to train them in observing and recording behavior.

Methods for dealing with extreme undesirable behavior or crisis situations were acted out and were discussed by the staff.

Emphasis was placed on how to talk to a child and how to find out the way the child saw the experience himself. Ways of preventing a crisis were introduced, e.g. when tension is building in the group, remove the child who seems to be the instigator or find an activity in which to involve the child that gets him away from the group.

Techniques of interviewing a child were discussed, with emphasis on helping the child to verbalize what he saw in a given situation following an event, on ways of getting information from a child, on speaking the language of a child, on how to show enthusiasm to a child, and on how to listen to a child. Particular attention was given to teaching the staff to avoid being conned by the child. Senior staff members modeled the skills required.

When talking about the individual child's program, it was possible to relate again to all other aspects of the training program.

Summary

The need for continuous training on the cottage cannot be emphasized enough. There must be experienced people who work directly with the child-care staff and who have enough contact with the children to model appropriate handling of the children. It is also important to involve the staff in changes in procedures, forms, and so forth.

The staff member had to learn to see himself as the initiator, i.e. as the person responsible for establishing a positive atmosphere and a positive relationship prior to the child's misbehavior. Staff had to be taught not to confront a child or to encounter a situation in such a way as to encourage a child to become defiant.

After the staff acquired some experience, the incidents that they had experienced were used as materials for ongoing training. As staff members developed their skills, they were given more and more opportunity to develop group activities, programs for individual children, and programs for the remediation of specific problems. Staff also were given opportunities to set up systems of recording progress in these programs.

Chapter 6

IMPLEMENTATION OF THE MILIEU PROGRAM

FROM THE start of the research project, children were housed in a new, single-level brick building, Cottage G, on the grounds of the Adler Zone Center. Cottage G (Fig. 3), which operated as a self-contained living unit, was one of three cottages at the Adler Zone Center. Each cottage had kitchen facilities, dining rooms, recreational areas, and office space, in addition to the children's rooms. Meals, other than breakfast, were not prepared at the cottage, but were delivered from the main Adler kitchen. The capacity of the cottage, as defined by the number of Adler staff and space, was 15 to 16 children. There were twelve bedrooms, a TV room, arts and crafts room, game room, and an activity room. The girls and younger boys were assigned rooms on one side of the courtyard and the older boys on the other. Open play areas surrounded Cottage G, and there were two outside areas with play equipment. The Adler Zone Center's school and a small gym were housed in a nearby building (Fig. 1).

Children who were admitted to the research-project cottage were accepted for a minimum stay of three months. After a child had been in residence for six weeks, a report was prepared for the Adler Zone Center's Clinical Review Committee; at that time, the length of stay was determined by them. Nine months was normally the maximum length of time that this committee would allow a child to stay. It was possible to request extensions as long as the total length of stay did not exceed one year.

Program Planning

Before a child entered the treatment program, one staff member was designated as that child's Intramural Counselor. Staff who were given the responsibility of being Intramural Counselors to children were experienced staff members and had college degrees

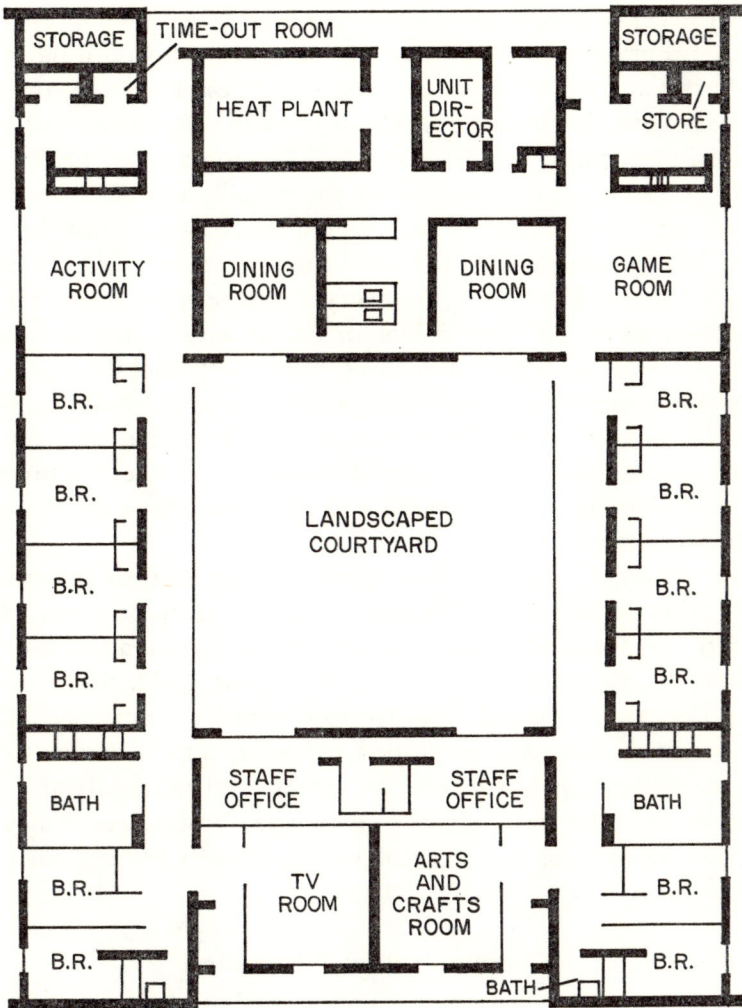

Figure 3. Floor plan of Cottage G.

or were close to receiving a college degree. Being an Intramural Counselor to a child meant that the staff member assumed certain important responsibilities (Appendix A) for planning that child's program and monitoring its implementation. Initially Intramural Counselors were supervised quite closely by the Project Director, Cottage Director, or Project Coordinator through regular weekly meetings. The continued development of each child's program was monitored by the Project Coordinator in collaboration with the Cottage Director. These two monitors met regularly with the Intramural Counselors to help them deal with any problems connected with the child's program; to review the child's progress on the cottage, in the school, and at home; and also to aid the Counselor in formulating future plans for the child. These sessions tended to function as ongoing training sessions for the Counselor. As everyone developed more experience, these meetings became less formal in nature, and the Intramural Counselor began assuming more responsibility for the planning of these programs. The procedure, as it finally evolved, usually consisted of the development of a tentative program by the Counselor, which he then discussed with the Extramural Case Coordinator, the teachers, and the research staff before it was implemented.

Intramural Counselors were given a great deal of latitude in developing the specific procedures used on each program. This allowed the Counselor the opportunity to be creative and innovative in the way that he planned for his child. Some of the first programs developed were quite dissimilar from each other. As more programs were developed, procedures used by one Counselor were frequently adopted by others, and gradually the programs grew to be more similar in nature. Procedures that were tried and found not to be useful were gradually eliminated from the programs.

Communication Channels

Communication among the staff was absolutely essential for the research project to be implemented effectively. Several different channels were routinely used to communicate information.

The Intramural Counselor was expected to meet at least weekly with the Extramural Case Coordinator to review the child's progress, to make adjustments in the treatment as needed, to coordinate home visits and the planning for continuity between the cottage and home programs. The amount of involvement that the Counselor had in planning and implementing the child's program in the home varied widely for the individual child, and it depended primarily upon how closely the Extramural Case Coordinator involved himself with the child's family. The Counselor also was expected to meet regularly with the child's schoolteachers and to aid in planning the child's program in the school.

Regular meetings were scheduled to provide a channel whereby staff could raise questions or seek solutions to problems related to the operation of the program. Decisions made at these meetings were communicated to all staff in the form of minutes taken during the meeting. Meetings, at which the entire staff was present, were held occasionally when there was a major change in cottage operation or when it was felt to be necessary from a training aspect. Similar meetings were held with school personnel.

The Project Director held monthly meetings with the Extramural Case Coordinators to keep them informed of the overall project activities and anticipated changes. These meetings offered opportunity for feedback to the research staff and training opportunities for the Extramural Case Coordinator.

Each child had a cardex, i.e. a folder in which cards were inserted in a staggered fashion allowing for rapid access to a given card, which contained all the information pertaining to a child's program. These cardexes were kept in a central location in the staff office and constituted the most complete and accurate source of information about a child's program. When a child began a new program, the Intramural Counselor was responsible for seeing that all the information was typed up and put in the cardex. A child's program was not begun until the cardex was complete. Whenever a new program was begun, a copy was also distributed to each staff member so that they could read their own copy rather than all having to read the cardex at one time.

Minor program changes occurred frequently with most children's programs. These changes were usually not extensive enough to necessitate a redistribution of the whole program to the staff. Communication of these changes were handled through "staff slips." A bulletin board in the staff office was blocked off into sections and each was labeled with the name of a child in the program. If a change was made in the child's program, the appropriate card in the cardex was changed to bring it up to date, and then a staff slip was put on the bulletin board under the child's name. This slip listed the names of the staff members, and a notation indicated the part of the program that had been changed. At the beginning of the shift, staff were expected to check the board for any new staff slips, and after they had read of the change in the cardex, they were to check off their names in order to indicate that they were aware of the change. These staff slips also were used to make sure that other important items of information were communicated to the staff. Any notice or memo that was posted for the staff had a staff slip attached. This proved to be a fairly effective way to make sure that the staff kept up with program changes.

Various memory aids were employed to make it easier for the staff to recall certain contingencies. For example, children on the response-cost punishment condition carried a yellow Mark Sheet, while those on time-out condition carried a white Mark Sheet. Information frequently used in certain places was posted in those locations for easy reference. For example, the number of marks each child paid for meals was posted next to the dining-room door. The Mark Sheets provided information regarding the child's program. If a worker was not certain about a child's targets, he could ask to see the Mark Sheet since the targets were indicated on each child's sheet.

Information that was not related to program changes but that needed to be communicated from shift to shift was written in a report book. Each staff member was expected to read this report book as soon as he started to shift.

Each child had a log book, and the staff on each shift were required to write a brief description of the child's behavior during that shift in the log book. This information was particularly useful to the Intramural Counselors and Extramural Case Coordinators, who wanted to know something of the child's behavior during the shifts when they were not present.

A data book for each child was kept in the staff office. This book was kept to provide the Intramural Counselor with information gathered concerning the child's behavior. This book contained (a) a daily summary of the number of marks earned by the child in each of his target areas, (b) a daily summary of how the child spent his marks, (c) a daily summary of punishable behavior, and (d) a weekly summary of the observation data gathered on the child's behavior on the unit.

For the purpose of emphasis, the following discussion on the implementation of the milieu program is subdivided into the cottage, school, and home programs. These three programs are not mutually exclusive, but rather they are overlapping aspects of the total program. The instructions that were given to the staff for implementing the program are in Appendix C, Procedures and Policies. More explicit examples of the implementation process are in Chapter 7, "Individual Programs."

Cottage Program

Each child's cottage program was based on the four levels described in Chapter 2, Dimension 1 and incorporated Dimensions 2, 3, 4, and 5.

Orientation Level. A child was placed on the Orientation Level as soon as he entered the cottage. The child remained on this level for a period of from one to three weeks before beginning the Level I program. The Orientation Level gave the staff an opportunity to assess the child's problem behaviors and behavioral deficits; to evaluate the child's strengths; to acquaint the child with the daily routine of the cottage; and to allow him a period to adapt. Thus, the staff had a chance to observe the child's more typical behavior patterns before the treatment program was begun.

On the Orientation Level, the child was given a Mark Sheet each day with enough marks on it to allow him access to all reinforcers available. This sheet was given to the child first thing in the morning, and the marks were negotiable for that day only. While on the Orientation Level, a child was not allowed to save marks from one day to the next. The child was allowed to spend these marks for any of the available backups, with the exception that home visits were not permitted during this period. Another restriction was that off-unit activities were limited to two per week, one on the weekends and one during the week. All privileges, such as snacks, weekly parties, and cold drinks, were purchased with these noncontingent marks.

Prices were arbitrarily set as five marks per item or event. Things that were rented for a period of time were generally five marks per half hour. The actual price charged a child was regarded as relatively unimportant since we were really interested in acquainting the child with the notion of exchanging marks for pleasurable things, and also in assessing which things a child would choose to take advantage of when they were available on a noncontingent basis.

During the Orientation Level, the frequency of the various behaviors defined as punishable (Chapter 2, Dimension 5) were recorded. No specified contingencies were employed for those punishable behaviors assigned to the 100 through 500 Levels. Staff members were allowed to use their own judgment in dealing with undesirable behaviors that were severely disruptive. Staff members were instructed to "do their own thing" in order to handle these situations. Punishable behaviors at the 600 and 700 Levels resulted in contingencies even during Orientation Level (Appendix C).

While the child was on the Orientation Level, his Intramural Counselor was instructed to spend as much time as possible with the child, getting to know him and observing his behavior in many different situations. The Counselor also was instructed to gather suggestions from other staff members regarding potential target behaviors. The Counselor was to gather the data collected on the child during Orientation Level, such as what reinforcers the child purchased with his marks, the child's performance of the behaviors on the Daily Checklist, and the frequency of the various categories of punishable behavior. Using these sources of data, the Counselor then was to prepare a proposed Level I program before a treatment planning meeting was held.

At some point during Orientation Level, a treatment planning meeting was held to develop and to specify the treatment program for that child. People at this meeting were the Intramural

Counselor, Extramural Cases Coordinator, Cottage Director, Project Director and/or Project Coordinator, and possibly other representatives of the research staff. The treatment plan that evolved during this meeting would specify the target behaviors that would be the focus of the Level I program. During this meeting, decisions were made regarding the child's daily earning power, specific target behaviors, i.e. appropriate social behaviors, and whatever minimum appropriate behaviors were deemed necessary. A list of backups that would be available to the child and the price of each one were also determined at this time. Specification was made of any special procedures or standing rules that would apply to this child while on this program. The criteria for movement to Level II was made as specific as possible in terms of what changes were expected and how they were to be evaluated. The original plan concerning movement from one level to the next was that the criteria for movement would be made quite specific and objective. This was achieved in some cases, but it was found that it was difficult to do with many children. If the target areas were broad categories rather than very specific behaviors, the criteria for movement was difficult to specify objectively and tended instead to be based more on the Intramural Counselor's subjective evaluation of gains rather than specific objective criteria. After the treatment program was formulated, the Intramural Counselor was responsible for seeing that it was typed and distributed to the staff and that the details of the program were explained to the child before it was put into effect.

Level I. The Level I program was seen as an introduction for the child to contingent reinforcement within a structured environment. Targets selected for this level were generally those that were felt to be easily modifiable and thus would give the child an opportunity to experience very quickly the positive consequences of changing or modifying his behavior. The length of time the child remained on a Level I program was determined individually and was based on changes in the child's behavior, but four to six weeks was the typical length of a Level I program.

When a child began a Level I program, he also began to experience systematic punishment contingencies (Appendix C).

Each child, when beginning a program, was assigned randomly to one of two punishment conditions, i.e. time out or response cost. The length of time that a child remained on a specific condition was determined by the stability of his punishable behavior. As soon as a stable effect was observed in response to the punishment procedures, a child was switched to the other punishment condition. This change was made quite independently of the child's promotion to another program level.

During the Level I program, the Intramural Counselor was responsible for communicating any changes to the rest of the staff and for monitoring them in their implementation of the program. Just prior to a child's promotion to Level II, a second treatment planning meeting was held. During this meeting, the targets and procedures for the Level II program were determined.

Level II. This level was established with the expectation that the bulk of the child's behavior changes would be made while on this level. Typically, there was not one program associated with Level II, but there were series of programs that were designated as Level II programs. When gains were made on an initial Level II program such that the Intramural Counselor felt that it was time to shift the program to other targets or to alter in some way the procedures being used, a new program would be developed. These programs were designated as Level II-Phase II, Level II-Phase III, and so on. They were different from the initial Level II programs, e.g. the emphasis placed on certain targets were changed, or some behaviors were shifted from mark reinforcement to Premack contingencies, or the number of marks used to reinforce certain categories might have been reduced.

At the point when the changes specified by the targets of the Level II programs had been made, a treatment planning meeting was again held to establish a Level III program for the child.

Level III. The major function of the Level III program was to phase the child off the mark system and to bring his behavior more directly under the control of social reinforcement and Premack management contingencies. While the number of marks being earned for various target behaviors might have been reduced on the Level II programs, the use of marks was usually quite minimal on a Level III program. The Level III program that was established for the child was to be as close as possible to a program that could be implemented in the home by the parents.

For most children, Level III was a time when they were spending less time on the cottage and more time in the home or public-school situation. With all children, efforts were made to work with the home or target placement to establish some kind of a system that would maintain the gains made at Adler. The nature and success of these efforts varied widely across the children.

When the level system was initially implemented (Chapter 2, Dimension 1), it called for a promotion ceremony or party to be held each time a child was promoted from one level to another. This was to call public attention to the child's achievement and to set up a situation in which he might receive a great deal of social reinforcement and recognition for his progress. These promotion parties or ceremonies gradually became less elaborate after the children became involved in the movement system.

Feedback and Reinforcement

After the three-week period on the Orientation Level when no systematic contingencies (positive or negative) were used in response to the child's behavior, the beginning of the child's Level I program marked the beginning of his treatment. The keystone to each child's program was to communicate systematically the expected behavior and positive consequences for the emission of these expected behaviors (Chapter 2, Dimensions 2, 3, 4). The child's program served as a guideline to the staff and indicated which behaviors were to receive positive attention. The vehicle used to systematize these positive consequences was the Mark Sheet (Chapter 4).

Marks were given to the child for the designated target behaviors throughout the entire day, whenever they were observed to occur. This required that the staff be continually sensitive to the occurrence of the child's target behaviors. Staff did not just stand around waiting for appropriate behavior to occur, but rather activities were planned that were apt to increase the probability of appropriate behavior. Staff were also encouraged to develop their own skills in eliciting positive behavior.

The fact that marks were given systematically, using a standard procedure, did not mean that marks were given in a mechanical, robot-like fashion. Staff were instructed to give social praise and approval at the same time that they were dispensing the mark. Social approval was not standardized but might take many forms, such as positive statements, smiles, and various sorts of physical contact. The development of warm personal relationships between the staff and children was in no way discouraged but was rather encouraged. By the time the child left the treatment program, it was expected that the major source of reinforcement maintaining the child's appropriate behavior would be positive social responses from the staff.

Staff were instructed to dispense the marks as soon after the emission of the behavior as possible. In some situations, there was delay in the delivery of the marks, since it was difficult and/or undesirable to interrupt some ongoing situation, such as a ball game, in order to give marks. When there was a delay of this sort, staff were instructed to provide feedback, as much as possible, i.e. a verbal description of the behavior for which the child was receiving the mark, e.g. "This is for picking up the bat and handing it to Johnny." Staff were also instructed to make a greater effort to dispense the marks immediately after the behavior with younger children or with a child who was relatively new in the program.

Positive feedback, i.e. a verbal description of the behavior, marks, and social approval, was given by the staff even when the children were off-unit. The nature of the activity, e.g. ice skating, swimming, movie, frequently made it necessary to delay the reinforcer until the completion of the activity. Punishable behavior on an off-unit activity was handled in several different ways. If the child was on the response-cost condition, he was fined in the usual manner. The way in which a time out was handled depended upon the nature of the situation. If it was possible, a child was taken out of earshot and required to sit facing away from the group. In other situations, a child was required to spend the allotted time sitting in the car by himself.

Precise scheduling of the marks, in terms of ratio or interval schedules, was not seen as practical since ten to twelve different staff might be involved with the child during the day. Thus, most marks were given on some sort of variable ratio or interval schedule. A few of the children's programs did attempt to specify the use of a particular interval schedule whenever the child was engaged in a certain kind of activity. Interval schedules were used rather consistently for giving marks within the school situation.

The Mark Sheet, which was carried daily by the child, served to systematize access to the reinforcers used as backups for the marks. Prices for the various backups for each child were established and were dependent upon his earning power. In setting prices, some consideration was given to determining the things a child really desired and the activities that the Intramural Counselor wanted the child to engage in. Thus, the price for TV might be set fairly high; the game room, which provided an opportunity for interaction, might be priced fairly low.

Marks earned by the child were exchanged for backups at various times during the day. Access to some backups, such as the activities of going off-unit, gym, and swimming, were purchased at certain times during the day. Other things, such as games, art supplies, and so forth, were available most times when a child might be free.

The procedure for indicating that marks had been exchanged for something was for a staff to draw a line through the marks being spent with the felt tipped pen attached to his marker. These pens and ink were a distinctive pink in color and children were not allowed access to pens of this color. After the staff member had marked out the marks being spent, he indicated what the child had purchased directly above the marks. Thus, the child's Mark Sheet provided information about the behaviors to be reinforced, how many marks were to be given for these behaviors, how many marks a child earned in each category for that day, which staff members had given him the marks, how many marks the child had spent, and for what he had spent them.

At the end of the day, the child submitted his Mark Sheet, and the information was recorded in each child's data book. Marks that were not spent were generally saved for future use, and each Mark Sheet had a space where savings could be recorded and accumulated. The programs of a few children did not allow them to save marks. This was done if the child was not spending or if it was felt that starting from zero each day was necessary in order to maintain the child's behavior.

A number of reinforcers constituted a standard list of backups that were routinely used for most children. Appendix C contains a sample list of backups. The program allowed for some flexibility regarding the use of idiosyncratic reinforcers. Practical limitations, such as money, staff time, and availability, governed the use of these idiosyncratic reinforcers. Examples of reinforcers that were used in this fashion included paying rent to keep a frog, paying to be with a group of older children, and paying to obtain special items of clothing.

Punishment

Two kinds of consequences were programmed to follow systematically those behaviors designated as undesirable or punishable (Appendix C, Punishment Contingencies). Two different punishment procedures were used in order to evaluate the relative effects of these two procedures upon undesirable behavior. Children were assigned on a random basis to one or the other of these procedures before they began their Level I program. After a stable effect was achieved as a result of the first procedure, the child was then switched to the second procedure. After a stable effect was observed in response to the second procedure, the Intramural Counselor was then allowed to decide which procedure he wished to continue using with the child's behavior. The two procedures were a form of time out and response cost.

Time out. Time out (TO) involved putting the child in an isolation room (a bare, tiled room, 3 × 5 × 10 feet, with a screened overhead light and a small Plexiglass window in the door) where he was required to spend a certain length of time. The length of time spent in this room depended upon which of the punishable behaviors the child had emitted. When the child committed a punishable behavior while on the time-out condition, he was told he must go to time out because of "X" behavior. A staff member accompanied the child to the room. If the child continued to emit the punishable behavior after being told he must go to time out, or if he emitted other punishable behaviors before reaching the time-out room, the time he was to spend in time out was increased by half. The length of time the child was required to serve was not begun if the child was having a tantrum, making noise, kicking, or in other ways being disruptive in the time-out room (Appendix C, "Time-out Procedures"). The use of physical force to take a child to time out was very aversive to the staff, especially if the child was older or very large. A procedure was developed, in response to this situation, which worked fairly well most of the time. After a child was told he must serve a period in time out and he refused to go, staff would tell him that his time would not start until he went to the time-out room. Then the staff ignored him and waited for him to indicate he was ready to start his time. If the child continued to be disruptive or attempted to engage in activities, then the staff would remove him physically.

Response cost. Response cost (RC) consisted of a procedure for fining a child in response to his emitting those behaviors defined as punishable. The amount of the fine depended on which of the behaviors the child had emitted and also on the child's earning power. When a child emitted a punishable behavior while on the response-cost condition, he was told that he would be fined "X" number of marks because of "X" behavior. If the behavior continued or if he emitted other punishable behavior, he was fined for each occurrence of any punishable behavior. For behaviors that were continuous in nature, such as defiance or a tantrum, it was necessary to define what constituted a single occurrence of this behavior. This was defined as a fifteen-second interval. Thus, if a child emitted a tantrum for two minutes, he was fined for eight instances of tantrums. If a child did not have enough marks to pay his fine, he went into debt and was not allowed to spend marks for any other purpose until the fine was paid (Appendix C, "Response-cost Procedures"). The accumulation of large debts became a problem with some children, and special procedures were developed to aid them in earning their way out of debt more quickly. These procedures are described in connection with the results of the punishment study (Chapter 8).

Seven levels of punishable behavior (Chapter 2, Dimension 5) were specified. These levels were ranked hierarchically in terms of staff ratings of the severity of the behavior on each level. Standard penalties were prescribed for the behaviors on the 100 through 500 Levels. Contingencies for those behaviors on the 600 and 700 Levels were determined individually for each child. Contingencies were not invoked for the behaviors at the 100 through 500 Levels during Orientation Level.

Time-out penalties were assigned to the behavior levels as follows:

>100 Level—10 minutes
>200 Level—20 minutes
>300 Level—30 minutes
>400 Level—40 minutes
>500 Level—50 minutes

The amount of response cost that was attached to each level of behavior depended on the earning power of the child. The mark fines for punishable behavior, based on the earning power per day were as follows:

Earning power of 1 to 50 marks
100 Level — 1 mark
200 Level — 2 marks
300 Level — 4 marks
400 Level — 8 marks
500 Level — 12 marks

Earning power of 51 to 85 marks
100 Level — 2 marks
200 Level — 4 marks
300 Level — 8 marks
400 Level — 16 marks
500 Level — 24 marks

Earning power of 86 to 115 marks
100 Level — 3 marks
200 Level — 6 marks
300 Level — 12 marks
400 Level — 24 marks
500 Level — 36 marks

Earning power of over 115 marks
100 Level — 4 marks
200 Level — 8 marks
300 Level — 16 marks
400 Level — 32 marks
500 Level — 48 marks

The results of comparison made between the use of these two procedures are discussed in Chapter 8.

Daily Schedule

Children were awakened at 7:45 A.M. each day. They were expected to dress, to make their beds, and to straighten up their rooms before breakfast was served at 8:15 A.M. The Adler Zone Center school day began at 9:00 A.M. Most children were scheduled for classes from 9:00 A.M. to 12:00 noon and 1:00 to 3:00 P.M. with maybe two half-hour periods free. These free periods were usually spent in some type of free play in the gym or outside. The school schedules for each child were quite varied from week to week. The schedule was altered to accommodate the scheduled one-to-one tutorial time or special activities, such as home economics, music, or shop, for each child. At 3:00 P.M., all children had a structured physical education (PE) period. Usually there was one PE activity for the girls and another for the boys. The organization of PE varied depending upon the composition of the cottage population at that time. After PE, children turned in their school Mark Sheets to staff, and cold drinks were served to those who had earned them. From roughly 4:15 P.M. until dinner, which was served at 5:00 P.M., children could spend their marks for various activities. TV and playing outside or in the activity room were always available at this time. Access to additional activity areas, such as the game room and the arts and crafts room, depended on whether there was enough staff to cover all these areas.

After dinner there was another activity period from 5:45 until 6:30 P.M. Outside activities, the game room, and the activity room were routinely available during this time. At 6:30 each evening, there was a forty-five-minute study hall. All children spent this time in one of the dining rooms engaged either in homework or in some form of quiet game activity. The evening schedule after study hall varied. Off-unit activities were offered routinely on two evenings each week, and every other week there was the possibility of an off-unit activity on a third evening. On evenings when there was an off-unit activity scheduled, study hall was only one-half hour long for those who were going off-unit. The off-unit activity began at 7:00 P.M. and typically lasted until 8:30. Those not going off-unit were allowed to buy things from the store from 7:15 to 7:30 P.M., and then were allowed access to outdoor activities or the activity room of the cottage if the weather was bad. Children under ten years of age, who did not go off-unit, showered from 8:00 to 8:30 P.M. Snacks were then served at 8:30 and the younger children went to bed at 9:00. Children who went off-unit showered from 9:00 to 9:30. Younger children who had been off-unit then went to bed at 9:30, and the older children had to be in their rooms at 9:30.

On evenings when there was not an off-unit activity scheduled, the store was open from 7:15 until 7:30. From 7:30 to 8:00, some sort of structured group activity was held, usually a form of group game. At 8:00, all children under ten showered, snacks were served at 8:30, and at 9:00 they went to bed. Older children showered from 9:00 to 9:30, and at 9:30 they were expected either to be in their rooms or in bed. Most children had the opportunity to earn staying up one-half hour later than their regular bedtime. If they earned this privilege, they had to be ready for bed and in their rooms, but they could read, play a quiet game, work on a model, and so forth. Appendix C contains a Daily Schedule of Activities.

The staff covered the cottage and functioned twenty-four hours a day, seven days a week. Two employees worked only the night shift from 11:00 P.M. to 7:30 A.M. All other staff worked both the day (7:30 A.M. to 3:30 P.M.) and the evening (3:00 P.M. to 11:00 P.M.) shifts. The staff routinely alternated working a week of the day shift followed by a week of the evening shift. The composition of the staff, in terms of male versus female, varied from time to time, but it usually was about 50-50. With the exception of the night shift, there were usually from four to six staff members scheduled on each shift.

Each staff member was expected to be thoroughly familiar with, and participate in, the implementation of the milieu program. All staff were expected to reinforce target behaviors, to invoke punishment contingencies, and record certain data. All staff were expected to provide models of appropriate behavior for the children and to relate to the children in a friendly, adult fashion. The teaching, direction, and supervision of play activities were also a routine part of all staff's jobs.

School Program

The child's Intramural Counselor and teachers determined the behaviors that were to be reinforced and the number of frequency with which the marks were to be given. The behavioral and academic guidelines remained very much the same although they were stated more explicitly for each child. School Mark Sheets were developed for each child that specified the child's targets and the number of marks to be given.

At the end of the school day, the child turned in his School Mark Sheet, and the marks earned in the classroom were converted into spendable marks. The number of spendable marks a child earned for his school performance was usually less than the number of school marks he received. A method of prorating the number of school marks was used because the actual number of school marks a child had an opportunity to earn each day varied widely with the school schedule. This also enabled the teacher to give marks fairly frequently without inflating the child's economy, e.g. if a child had an opportunity on a given day to earn 50 school marks and he earned 45 of them, he would have earned 90 percent of the number of spendable marks assigned to his school performance; if the number of spendable marks assigned to his school earning was 20, then he would have earned 18 spendable marks.

The punishment contingencies used in the classroom were almost identical to those used on the cottage. In addition to the standing rules that applied to the classroom, cheating was indicated as a punishable behavior on the 200 Level. All punishable behaviors occurring in the classroom resulted in a time-out contingency. The pilot punishment study which used the response-cost procedure in the classroom, indicated that it was too difficult to administer consistently in this situation. Children emitting a punishable behavior in the classroom were sent from the room by the teacher. A child-care worker would then take the child to the time-out room. If the time to be served was twenty minutes or less, the child was taken to a time-out room in the school building. If the time to be served was more than twenty minutes, the child was taken then to the cottage time-out room.

When a number of new teachers entered the Adler School, it was felt that the presence of a cottage staff member would be useful in helping the teacher implement the program. It was arranged with the Adler School that the cottage staff would sit in the two classrooms that contained most of the children from the project cottage. These staff were to give marks for social behavior and also were to invoke the punishment contingencies. The teachers were to give marks for academic behavior. The teachers were also to cue the cottage staff if the teacher felt that the child was being defiant or had violated a classroom rule and should be removed.

Integration of the child back into the public-school classroom was the ultimate goal for every child. The Extramural Case Coordinator and Intramural Counselor were expected to work with the Adler teacher to accomplish this goal. Usually the first step was the establishment of communication, between the Adler teacher and the public-school teacher, about the materials used and the achievement required in the public-school classroom. Public-school teachers were encouraged to visit the Adler School in order to observe the child there. Sometimes this was the most that could be accomplished with a given child's case. If the public school the child was to attend was close enough, he might start attending public school for part of the day before he was released from Adler. Some children were placed part time in local schools, even though they were ultimately returning to schools in other communities. This arrangement was not always possible for out-of-town children, and another strategy consisted of having the child attend his own school one or two days a week (usually a Friday and/or a Monday) in conjunction with his weekend visit home. Arrangements for teacher visits, communication of information, and part-time attendance were made whenever possible. When a child attended a public school on a part-time basis, a plan was generally established with the public-school teacher, whereby a rating of various behaviors was made by the teacher. Various backups within the cottage program would then be made contingent upon these ratings. If possible, this method of backing up public-school performance was shifted from the cottage to the home when the child was discharged. In a few cases, the target placement was so tenuous that little or no planning could be done regarding school placement. In these cases, the Extramural Case Coordinator made arrangements to work with the public school in order to deal with the child in the manner that would most effectively maintain the gains made at Adler.

Home Program

During the period the child spent on the Orientation Level, he was not allowed to make home visits. As soon as the Level I program began, home visits were possible and were regarded as an important part of the child's program. The only children for whom home visits were not programmed were those children who were under the guardianship of a state agency and, therefore, were not being returned to their families. Seven of the thirty children serviced by this program were in this category. Two of these were placed in foster homes. As soon as these homes were identified, the children began making home visits. The other five children were placed in children's homes. When it was practical, weekend visits were arranged with the institution and were planned into fit the child's overall program.

The frequency, length, and structure of the home visits varied according to (a) practical considerations, such as distance and transportation; (b) the progress of work with the family; (c) the child's progress on the unit; and (d) the targets of the child's current program. The child's Extramural Case Coordinator was responsible for seeing that the family received help while the child was at Adler. In some cases, an Extramural Case Coordinator provided direct service and did all the therapeutic work with the family himself. In other cases, the Extramural Case Coordinator arranged for a community agency to provide some service, while he dealt with the family regarding specific arrangements, such as transportation and school placement.

The most effective method for working out home programs, which provided the most continuity between the cottage program and what happened while the child was at home, seemed to result when the Extramural Case Coordinator and Intramural Counselor worked together, with the family, in setting up the home program. Ideally the parents would be instructed in the basic principles of this research project (Chapter 2) before the child made any visits home. If possible, the parents might practice implementing these principles by setting up a program for other children still in the home. Then, a simple program might be worked out for the child's first visit home that would require the parents to identify the occurrence of some appropriate behavior and to follow it with some kind of positive consequence. As the parents gained more success and experience in implementing such contingencies, more behaviors might be added, and, if necessary, some sort of negative contingency might be incorporated to handle unacceptable behavior. This ideal was achieved with some cases but only approximated with others.

Home programs were usually tied to the cottage program in several ways. They frequently were used as reinforcers and were made contingent upon the performance of some behavior on the cottage. The behaviors, which the parents were instructed to reinforce, were the same behaviors that were identified as targets in the cottage program. The method used to reinforce these behaviors usually paralleled that in the cottage program, although the home programs were never as complex and frequently made more use of Premack contingencies. Some consistent form of punishment was often set up in the home. Whether response cost or time out was chosen usually depended on the parent's preference, plus considerations such as the availability of a room suitable for time out. Sometimes the home programs were set up so that a child's behavior during his weekend visit would elicit certain reinforcers on the unit. Occasionally, the program was set up so that a child's performance during one weekend visit would determine whether or not a visit was allowed the following weekend.

Monitoring the parent's progress in implementing such programs was one problem that was frequently encountered. In some cases, parental report that was based on the use of a behavior checklist was the only way to monitor home visits. A more effective way involved visits to the home, while the child was visiting, by either the Extramural Case Coordinator, Intramural Counselor, or a trained home intervener (a person who went into the home to help parents develop more effective management techniques). While this was more effective, it was often not practical because of staff shortages and the distances involved.

Another source of difficulty in implementing effective home programs was the motivation of parents to be actively involved in the child's program. While a verbal commitment was required in most cases before a child was admitted to Adler, this frequently did not equal a behavioral commitment.

Chapter 7

INDIVIDUAL PROGRAMS

Detailed descriptions of the programs for three of the thirty children who resided in the research-project cottage are provided as examples of some of the individual programs used. These three cases were selected to provide a representative cross section of the population serviced by the research project. Variables that were considered in the selection were age, sex, race, intellectual level, and type of presenting problem. These cases are being presented neither as the most successful among the programs nor as representing the complete range of procedures used in connection with the various programs. These cases do provide a sample of the various kinds of programs developed in response to the range of children admitted to the research project.

Appendix D contains a sample Mark Sheet and the cardex material for one child's program at all levels. Brief descriptions of the programs that were used with the remaining twenty-seven children are given in Appendix E.

SUBJECT 10

Presenting Problems

Subject 10 (C.B.) is a twelve-year-old black, retarded female, who was referred for treatment because of problems in school.

She had been placed in a trainable mentally handicapped classroom, where her academic work had been regressing. The teacher described C.B. as being isolative in the classroom and either refusing to speak or communicating in a soft, breathy whisper. These isolative behaviors did not interfere with her peer relations as she was described as playing and relating well to other children.

Her family consists of her unmarried mother and two older sisters, one of whom has a child and is living in the home. The mother does not work and has a history of illness.

Individual Programs

Cottage and School Programs

During the three-week orientation period, C.B. was observed to be very quiet, rarely speaking above a whisper. It was observed that she talked more readily to other children than to staff. She was hesitant to initiate contacts with other children, although she readily joined in if another initiated the contact.

Level I

Appropriate social behaviors. Three categories of social behavior were identified as targets on this program. These were as follows:

> Answering adults — 40 marks
> Answering children — 15 marks
> General — 15 marks

The emphasis of this program was upon her communicating verbally with adults. The 40 marks in the "Answering adults" category were given for single word verbalization directed at or in response to an adult. If the verbalization was more than one word, an additional mark was given. Marks in the "Answering children" category were given for verbalizations directed at or in response to a child. The "General" category was used to reinforce any generally appropriate social behavior, but emphasis was given to interactive behaviors.

Minimum appropriate behaviors. During the orientation period, C.B.'s performance of the routine self-care behaviors was observed to be quite high. It was therefore decided that no systematic contingencies would be needed for these behaviors.

School. Twenty spendable marks were given for the performance of appropriate social and academic behaviors in the classroom. During each half-hour class, C.B. could earn 3 school marks for social behavior, such as sitting at her desk, being on task, and answering when called upon, and 3 school marks for academic behaviors, such as task completion, neatness, and accuracy.

Punishment. C.B. was assigned initially to the response-cost punishment condition. Since her earning power was 90 marks per day, fines for the 100, 200, 300, 400, and 500 Levels of punishable behavior were 3, 6, 12, 24, and 36 marks, respectively. She remained on this condition for four weeks before being switched to time-out punishment. She was on the response-cost condition during the entire time she was on Level I.

Length of program. After two weeks on this program, there was a sufficient increase in the frequency and audibility of her verbalizations to warrant progression to a Level II program. Her attainment of this goal was rewarded by allowing her to keep a pair of gerbils in her room.

Level II

Appropriate social behaviors. Five categories of social behavior were labeled as targets on this program. They were as follows:

> Answering adults — 25 marks
> Answering children — 15 marks
> Spontaneous speech — 25 marks
> Loud talk — 5 marks
> General — 15 marks

To earn a mark in the "Answering adults" category, C.B. was required to answer with more than one word. On Level I a single word was sufficient for a mark. Marks in the "Answering children" category were given for verbalizations directed to another child. The 25 marks in the "Spontaneous speech" category were used to reinforce verbalizations that C.B. initiated. C.B. earned marks in the "Loud talk" category if her verbalizations were louder than the average person's speaking tone, i.e. if she shouted. Marks in the "General" category continued to be given for any generally appropriate social behavior.

Minimum appropriate behaviors. No systematic reinforcement was given for the performance of these behaviors.

School. C.B. continued to earn 20 spendable marks per day for appropriate school behavior. The procedure was the same as it was for Level I.

Punishment. After C.B. had been on her Level II program for two weeks, she was switched from response cost to time out. She remained on the time-out condition for the rest of her stay in the treatment program.

Special procedures. It had been noted on Level I that C.B. responded very well to earning badges, stars, and so forth. Hence, it was set up so that if she earned all the marks possible on the cottage, she would receive a large colorful badge to wear. For "loud talk" in the classroom, she earned special red stars that could be exchanged for a cold drink.

Length of program. After four weeks on this program, it was felt that it should be modified.

Level II—Phase II

Appropriate social behaviors. Two categories of social behavior were identified as targets on this program. They were as follows:

Talking — 20 marks
Group interaction — 20 marks

Marks in the "Talking" category were given for spontaneous speech, loud speech, and talking with adults. The marks in the "Group interaction" category were given if she joined a group of 2 or more children or if she was interacting with one other child as long as it was not M.D. At this point in her program, C.B. was spending most of her time with M.D., who was identified as her "boyfriend." For this reason, marks were not given when just the two of them were interacting.

Minimum appropriate behaviors. None of the self-care behaviors received any systematic contingencies.

School. Ten spendable marks were available for appropriate school behaviors. The procedure was the same as that described for Level I.

Punishment. C.B. was assigned to the time-out condition during the time she was on Level II-Phase II.

Length of program. C.B. remained on Level II-Phase II for the rest of the time she was in the treatment program. Six weeks after beginning this program, she left for an extended home visit. After several weeks at home, she made several overnight visits to the cottage and was subsequently discharged.

Home Program

During C.B.'s stay at Adler she made frequent weekend home visits. When her Level II program began, a structured program for her home visits was initiated. A form was sent home each time C.B. made a visit, asking her mother to record C.B.'s performance of routine behaviors, such as taking care of her room and clothes, brushing her teeth and washing her hands, and being on time for meals. Ratings were to be made each day of the frequency of C.B.'s verbalizations, along with information that identified the situations in which she seemed to be the most and least verbal. The mother was instructed to give C.B. a mark when C.B. initiated a conversation or answered a question with more than one word. C.B. could earn up to 25 marks per day for these behaviors. Marks that were earned during the visit were exchanged for spendable marks on a 5 to 1 ratio and could be spent the next week.

Before C.B. was discharged, a student social worker was assigned to work with the mother. The student social worker frequently observed in the home and worked with the mother to help her to develop more consistent child-management techniques. These visits continued for several months after C.B. was discharged from the cottage program.

Data

Independent Observations

Cottage. C.B.'s observed deviant behavior decreased even though it was initially quite low (Fig. 4).

The percentage of the time C.B. was observed to be engaging in verbal behavior is of interest, since this was the primary target on all her programs (Fig. 5). The data does indicate a definite increase in occurrence of verbal behavior observed during the Orientation Level.

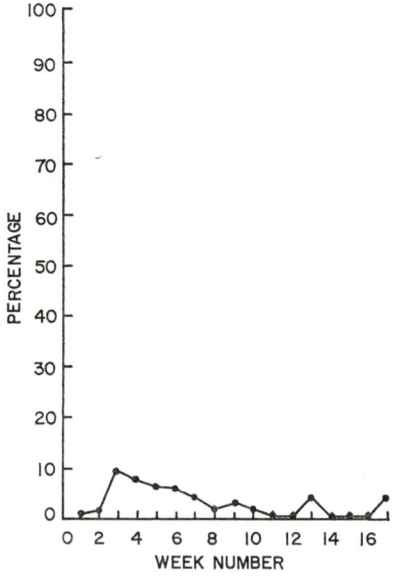 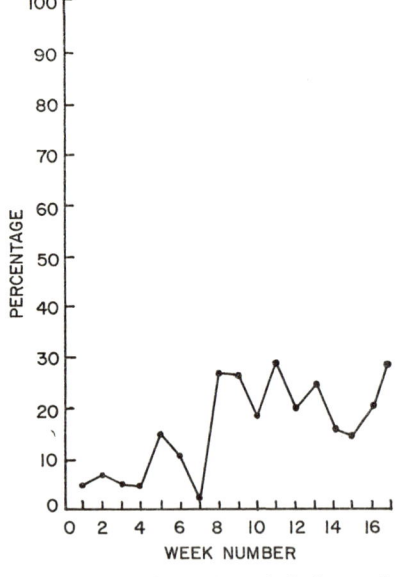

Figure 4. Subject 10, unit independent observations, percentage of deviant behavior.

Figure 5. Subject 10, unit independent observations, percentage of positive verbal behavior.

C.B. also received reinforcement for interacting, and the percentage of her interactions with others that were judged positive showed a consistent increase over the Orientation Level.

School. Observations in the school indicated a definite increase in verbal behavior (Fig. 6). Deviant behavior was initially quite low, but an increase was observed after her Level I program began. This increase persisted until Level II-Phase II began. At that point, deviant behavior returned to its original low frequency.

Daily Checklist

C.B.'s rate of performance of the MABs remained very high throughout her stay on the cottage, even though these behaviors were not ever reinforced with marks. It appears that these behaviors were well established when she entered the program, and the cottage routine and the social reinforcement present were adequate to maintain these behaviors.

Punishment Data

During baseline, C.B. exhibited a relatively low frequency (average of 2.8 incidents per day) of those behaviors that would result in the invoking of a punishment contingency.

When her program began, she was put on response-cost punish-

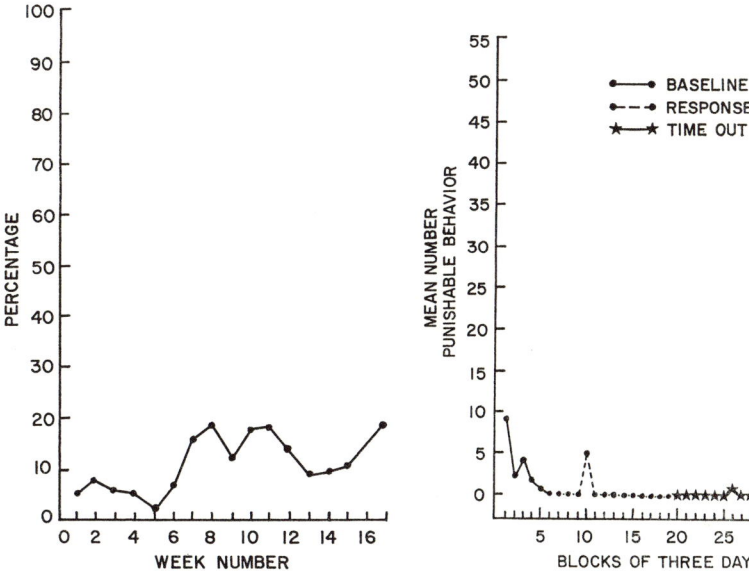

Figure 6. Subject 10, school independent observations, percentage of positive verbalizations.

Figure 7. Subject 10, frequency of punishable behavior.

ment. While on response cost, the incidence of her punishable behavior dropped to an average of .4 incidents per day. During the last few weeks on response cost, the frequency of punishable behavior dropped to zero.

The overall incidence of punishable behavior while on time out was even lower than during response cost (average of .03 incidents per day). The rate was also reduced to zero for the last few weeks of the time-out condition (Fig. 7).

SUBJECT 19

Presenting Problems

Subject 19 (H.L.) is an eleven-year-old black male of normal intelligence with a history of asthma and allergies, who was referred for treatment because of problems in both the home and school.

H.L. was characterized as always having had problems in school and never having had much academic success. He had difficulties getting along with his peers, picking fights and being verbally abusive. He reportedly spent much of his time in the classroom daydreaming, drawing pictures, or disturbing other children. He occasionally engaged in bizarre attention-getting behaviors, such as running to the board, drawing a funny design, then returning to his seat. Just prior to his admission, he had been expelled from a parochial school because of his aggressive outbursts toward other children.

His family consists of his parents and three sisters, one of whom was older. H.L. reportedly had some difficulty relating to his sisters, seeing them as picking on him. His main difficulties in the home were described as several incidences of petty theft and running away. His running away was reportedly done to avoid punishment from the father who was characterized as a harsh disciplinarian.

Cottage and School Programs

During the two-week Orientation Level on the cottage, H.L. was observed to lack skills in relating to other children. He showed a rather high incidence of such behaviors as assault on other children, destruction of other children's property, and defiance of adult requests. During this period, he averaged 46 punishable behaviors per day.

Level I

Appropriate social behaviors. Three categories of social behavior were identified as targets on this program. They were as follows:

Being nice to other kids — 25 marks
Cooperation — 5 marks
General — 10 marks

The "Being nice to kids" category was used to reinforce any kind of positive interaction that occurred between H.L. and at least one other child. Marks in the "Cooperation" category were used to reinforce compliance with staff requests and acceptance of limits. The "General" category was used to reinforce positive interactions with staff and constructive behaviors such as doing homework.

Minimum appropriate behaviors. H.L. did not receive marks for any of the MABs, but he earned the privilege of staying up one-half hour later than the regular bedtime, by performing 10 out of 11 designated self-care behaviors (Appendix D).

School. H.L. was able to earn 20 spendable marks for the performance of academic and appropriate social behaviors in school. During each half hour of class, he was able to earn 3 school marks for academic behavior, such as task completion, neatness, and accuracy, and 3 for social behavior, such as sitting at desk and being on task. If he earned at least 18 of the spendable marks available for school, he received a cold drink after school.

Punishment. H.L. was initially assigned to the response-cost punishment condition. His fines, as determined by his daily earning power, were 2, 4, 8, 16, and 24 marks for the 100, 200, 300, 400, and 500 Levels of punishable behavior. H.L. remained on the response-cost condition throughout his Level I program.

Special procedures. A special contingency was used in connection with weekend home visits. If H.L. committed any of those behaviors defined as most punishable (assault on an adult, AWOL, entering the staff office), he lost the privilege of a home visit for that weekend.

Length of program. H. L. was on this program (Appendix D) for seven weeks before beginning his Level II program.

Level II

Appropriate social behaviors. The focus of H.L.'s program continued to be upon positive peer interactions. The same categories of social behaviors that were targets on Level I continued to be targets on this program. The categories were as follows:

  Being nice to other kids — 15 marks
  Cooperation — 10 marks
  General — 10 marks

These categories were used to reinforce the same kinds of behaviors as were described on Level I, but on this program, the number of marks used for "Being nice to kids" category was decreased, while the number of marks for "Cooperation" was increased.

Minimum appropriate behaviors. None of the self-care behaviors had any systematic contingencies on this program.

School. The number of marks H.L. earned in school was reduced to 15 spendable marks, and in order to have a cold drink after school, he had to earn at least 13 of these marks. School marks were given in the same manner as described for Level I.

Punishment. H.L. continued on the response-cost condition during his Level II program.

Special procedures. On this program, H.L. was given the job of cleaning up the TV and activity rooms each day. He was able to earn 5 marks for the performance of this job. Special procedures concerning daily earning of marks and the payment of fines were also used on this program. If H.L. earned 57 or more marks and had no fines for that day, he received a star on his "Great Day Chart." When he had accumulated four such stars, he was allowed to go on a special off-unit activity with his Intramural Counselor.

At the time this program began, H.L. had accumulated a large debt from having been fined for punishable behavior. A special procedure was used to allow him to work himself out of debt so that he would once again be able to experience some payoff for good behavior. If he had a day where he had been fined less than 5 marks, 250 marks were subtracted from his debt; and for each consecutive day that he had less than 5 marks in fines, he was able to substract double the amount subtracted the day before. If he had a day when he was not fined at all, he was allowed to spend any marks he earned the next day, even though he may have still had a debt and ordinarily would not have been able to spend until it was completely eliminated. These procedures were set up to give him some incentive to go for longer periods of time without misbehaving.

Length of program. This program (Appendix D) was in effect for six weeks before a modification designated as his Level II-Phase II program began.

Level II — Phase II

Appropriate social behaviors. Four categories of social behavior were identified as targets on this program. These were as follows:

> Being nice to kids — 10 marks + plus points
> Cooperation — 10 marks + plus points
> General — 5 marks
> Being responsible about allergies — 10 marks + plus points

The "Nice to kids" category continued to be used to reinforce positive peer interactions.. The number of marks that could be earned was reduced, but he was able to earn additional marks in the form of plus points. Plus points were given just as marks were, but they did not figure into the regular economy in the same way as marks. They could not be spent for the regular backups, but they were saved instead toward a special activity with his Counselor. In order for H.L. to earn a "Compliance" mark on this program, he had to comply immediately and without grumbling or pouting. Marks in the "General" category were given for joining groups and participating in activities. The category labeled "Being responsible about his allergies" was used to reinforce taking medication, watching his diet, and taking the responsibility for sitting out of activities if he started to wheeze.

Minimum appropriate behaviors. No systematic contingencies were used for the performance of self-care behaviors.

School. The number of spendable marks that he could earn in school was increased to 20, and he was able to earn a cold drink if he received 17 of these marks. Otherwise the school program was the same as the previous program.

Punishment. H.L. continued to be on response-cost punishment during his Level II-Phase II program.

Special procedures. He continued to have the job of picking up TV and activity room, and its performance was reinforced by a snack at bedtime.

Special procedures were used to earn the weekly cottage party and special off-unit trips. H.L. was required to earn at least 40 marks, for two out of three days, in order to go to the cottage party. If he earned at least 53 marks, he was given a "Great Day" star; and after he had accumulated four stars, he was taken on a special off-unit trip by his Intramural Counselor.

Length of program. The Level II-Phase II program (Appendix D) was in effect for four weeks before he began a new program designated as his Level II-Phase III.

Level II — Phase III

Appropriate social behaviors. This program was set up to begin phasing H.L. out of the mark system. Four categories of social behavior were identified as targets. These were as follows:

      Good interaction with peers
      Cooperation
      Good conversation with staff
      Managing his allergies

There was no set number of marks that could be earned in any of these categories, but staff was instructed to continue reinforcing H.L. at approximately the same rate as on his previous program. While the labels of the categories were somewhat changed, basically the same behaviors that were reinforced on previous programs were also reinforced here.

Minimum appropriate behaviors. As on the previous programs no systematic contingencies were used for these behaviors.

School. He continued to earn 20 spendable marks in school as on his other programs, but now he was required to earn 18 in order to receive a cold drink after school.

Punishment. When H.L. began this program, all punishment contingencies were removed for a two-week period. At the end of this time, the time-out procedure was begun.

Special procedures. H.L. continued to have the job of straightening up the TV and activity rooms, which enabled him to earn staying up an extra half hour. Taking a shower was rewarded, on this program, by a bedtime snack.

The primary difference between this program and the preceding ones was the way in which H.L. spent his marks for the various reinforcers. Rather than spend the marks as he earned them for each reinforcer, he was required to pay a fixed sum once a week, which was called "rent." Paying "rent" would give him access to all reinforcers for the whole week. He was charged 45 marks per day for each full day he was on the cottage. He paid on Friday for the number of days he had spent on the cottage, and this gave him free access to all reinforcers for the next week. If he was not able to meet the amount of rent required, he lost a certain number of privileges for the whole week. How many and which privileges he lost were determined by the number of marks he was short. For example, if he was short 10 marks, he lost access to the store; but if he was short between 11 and 20 marks, he lost access to the store and the game room. Any marks that were left over after paying rent were applied toward a special off-unit activity with his Intramural Counselor.

Length of program. H.L. remained on this program (Appendix D) for five weeks before beginning his Level III program.

Level III

Appropriate social behaviors. On this program, H.L. ceased earning marks for good behaviors, but he continued to receive frequent social reinforcement. All activities in the program were made contingent upon generally good behavior, i.e. if he was not being appropriate, he was either denied access to an activity or else asked to leave activities he was already engaged in.

Minimum appropriate behaviors. No systematic contingencies were used with these behaviors.

School. H.L. no longer earned marks for appropriate school behaviors.

Punishment. Time-out punishment procedures were continued on the Level III program. He remained on time out for the rest of his stay in the treatment program.

Special procedures. Several specific contingencies were used on this program. Having two TO's in school was reinforced by a cold drink after school, less than two TO's during the day was backed up by a snack at bedtime, and staying up late was contingent upon having taken a shower.

Length of program. H.L. remained on this program (Appendix D) for the rest of the time he was in the treatment program. Because of illness and extended visits at home, he spent only nine days on the cottage while this program was in effect.

Home Program

During H.L.'s Level I program, home visits were rather infrequent, since there were some problems arranging for transportation. H.L. was from a city 75 miles from the Adler Zone Center. Only two home visits were made during the seven weeks on Level I. After his Level II program began, arrangements were made that allowed him to go home on the train, and from this point on, home visits were much more frequent. A Home Visit Form (Appendix D) was sent home with H.L. to elicit information from the parents regarding the weekend visit, i.e. what things went well, what problems occurred, how they handled them. The parents were also to record whether he performed certain behaviors, such as making his bed, brushing teeth, picking up his room, and taking a shower. The information from this form was used to assess his weekend visits, and if they had gone well, he received a free off-unit activity plus a discount on the price of his next home visit.

Progress in setting up a program of contingencies with the parents was hampered by several factors. One of the biggest problems was the limited accessibility of the parents. Both worked and the father was only in the home on weekends. This presented a problem in that the staff assigned to the case found it difficult to meet with or work with the parents. Aside from this difficulty, there was a basic conflict between the parents. This conflict concerned the father's absence from the home and the parent's individual ideas regarding discipline and child-rearing methods. All these factors combined to hamper the efforts that were made to develop a home program. A student social worker met with the mother on several occasions, in an effort to acquaint her with some of the basic principles of behavior modification. While there was some progress with this, the social worker felt that the effect of these sessions upon the mother's child-management behavior would be minimal.

After H.L. began his Level II-Phase III program, the home visits were lengthened to enable him to spend the weekend at home and then to spend first one day and then two days in public school before returning to the cottage. This was done to ease the transition from the Adler school back into the regular classroom.

Data

Independent Observations

Cottage. During H.L.'s Level I program, deviant behavior was observed to increase over the Orientation Level. After his Level II program began, there was a decrease in the percentage of deviant behavior. This decrease was maintained until his Level III program began, with the exception of one week during the period when the punishment contingencies were removed (Fig. 8).

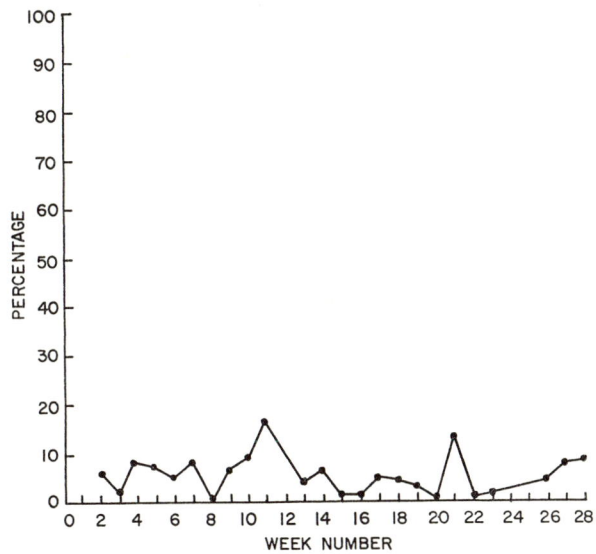

Figure 8. Subject 19, unit independent observations, percentage of deviant behavior.

Since much emphasis was placed on positive interaction, observer data pertaining to interactive behavior is of interest. The percentage of his interactions with peers and staff, which were observed to be positive, was quite high during Orientation Level. This generally high rate was maintained through most of his Level I program, but tapered off some toward the end and during the first week of the Level II program. During the rest of the Level II program, the high percentage of positive interactions was maintained. A slightly lower percentage of positive interactions was observed during the three weeks that he was on his Level III program (Fig. 9).

School. In the school, the percentage of deviant behavior showed an initial decrease over the rate that was observed before his progam began, although there were two weeks toward the end of his Level I program when there was a slight increase over the percentage of deviant behavior observed during Orientation Level. During his Level II program, which started during the three-week school vacation, there was a considerable drop in deviant behavior. This decrease was maintained until his last two weeks in the program, when there was an abrupt increase (Fig. 10).

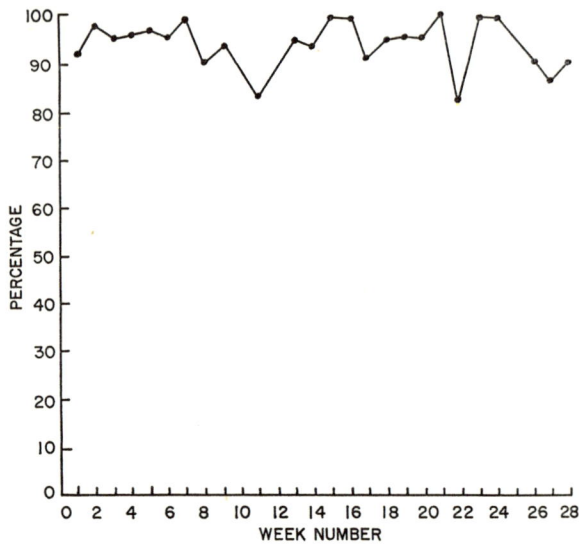

Figure 9. Subject 19, unit independent observations, percentage of positive interactions.

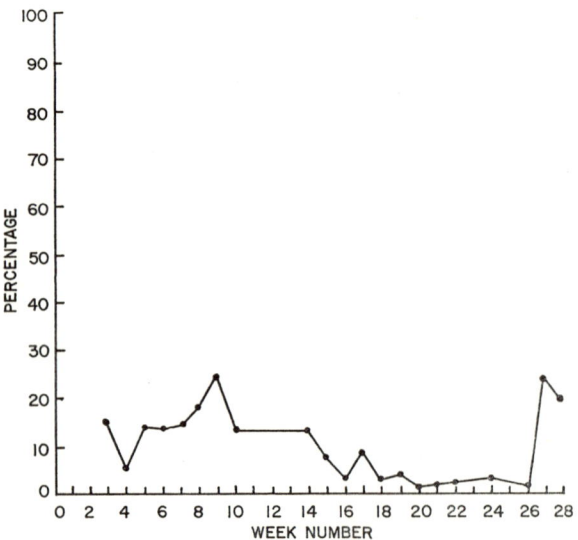

Figure 10. Subject 19, school independent observations, percentage of deviant behavior.

The percentage of his interactions in the classroom, which were observed to be positive, showed a sharp increase when his program began. With the exception of the last week on Level I, this increase showed a general decline throughout his Level I program. During Level II, an increase was again observed; and it was maintained until his last two weeks in the program, when there was an abrupt drop in postive interactions (Fig. 11).

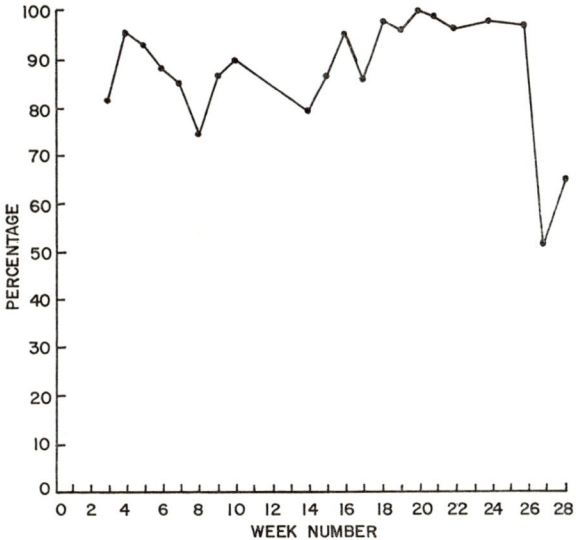

Figure 11. Subject 19, school independent observations, percentage of positive interactions.

Daily Checklist

Those behaviors that never received any systematic contingencies decreased slightly when H.L.'s program first began, but then returned to their previous frequency. Performance of these behaviors dropped off again during the last few weeks of the program.

A group of the Daily Checklist behaviors, i.e. bed made, room neat, dressed neat, and hands washed before lunch and dinner, teeth brushed after lunch and dinner, closets and drawers neat, and laundry put out, resulted in a Premack contingency during his Level I program. After the program began, there was an initial increase followed by a decrease in the performance of these behaviors. There was, however, an increase during the last three weeks of Level I to a rate well above that observed during Orientation Level. At that point, Premack contingencies were discontinued, and the performance of these behaviors generally decreased.

Punishment Data

During Orientation Level, H.L. exhibited a relatively high frequency (average 46 incidents per day) of behaviors for which punishment contingencies were invoked in the program. His most frequent category of punishable behavior was that labeled defiance, i.e. noncompliance. There was also a relatively high frequency of assault on other children and destructive behavior. There was a considerable decline in the frequency of punishable behavior during the last three days of the Orientation Level.

Institution of the response-cost procedures led to an immediate

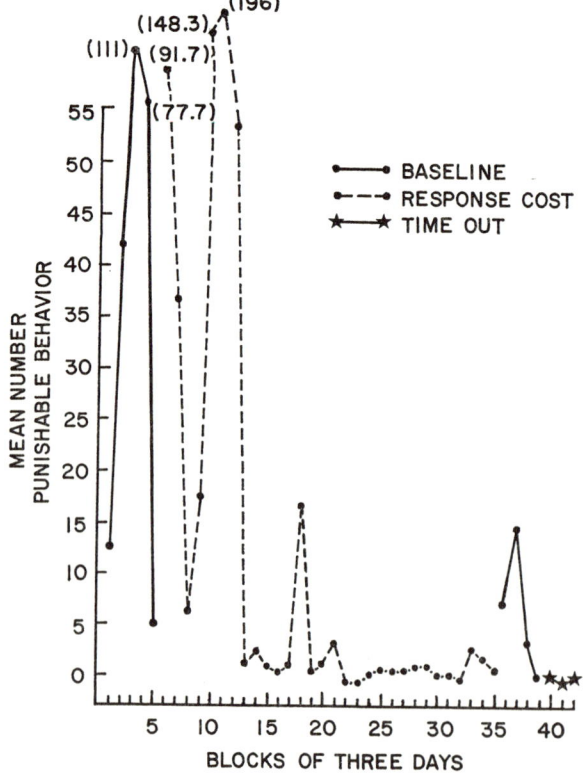

Figure 12. Subject 19, frequency of punishable behavior.

and dramatic increase in the rate of punishable behavior. During the first twenty-one days of response cost, the rate of punishable behavior was quite variable with several periods of extremely high rates. This was followed by a dramatic decrease to almost a zero rate, which was maintained for sixty-nine days, with the exception of a three-day period when there was a moderate increase (Fig. 12).

Before time-out procedures were begun, all punishment contingencies were suspended for a two-week period. There was an immediate increase in punishable behavior, but this increase was considerably lower than the frequency observed during Orientation Level (average frequency was 5.9 punishable behaviors per day). Before the two weeks were over, there was a decrease to approximately the rate observed during response-cost conditions. This low rate of punishable behavior continued after the time-out punishment was begun. Because of illness and extended home visits, H.L. was only on the cottage for nine full days while the time-out conditions were in effect. The average frequency of punishable behavior during the time-out condition was .4 incidents per day.

SUBJECT 21

Presenting Problems

Subject 21 (D.L.) is an eight-year-old white, functionally retarded male, who was referred for treatment because of problems in both the home and the school.

D.L. was not accepted for first grade because of his hyperactive behavior and inability to cooperate in a group setting. He had attended both Head Start and kindergarten for a short period of time. In those situations, he was described as being uncooperative with the teachers and was cooperative only in activities that he liked and then only for a short period of time. It was also noted that he had a speech problem in that he stuttered and stammered.

His family consists of his mother and father, both of whom are in the home. His father is retired, has had eye surgery, and his vision is seriously impaired. They live on his disability pension, and as a result, their financial resources are quite meager. The parents described D.L. as being "in and out of everything" with a very short attention span. They reported that he did not listen to what they told him and that attempts by them to discipline or punish him had been unsuccessful. D.L. had become more of a problem to them because he was getting older and larger.

Cottage and School Programs

During the first three days of a three-week Orientation Level, D.L. was observed to be very hyperactive, running from place to place and not remaining with any activity for more than a few minutes. This hyperactivity decreased after the first few days, but continued to be a problem. He had a great deal of difficulty following the daily schedule and performing routine self-care behaviors. He was also frequently defiant and exhibited many immature, dependent behaviors. Stuttering was also observed to be a problem.

Level I

Appropriate social behaviors. Three categories of social behavior were identified as targets on this program. They were labeled as follows:

> Mealtime behavior — 20 marks
> Grownup suggestions — 15 marks + plus points
> General — 10 marks + plus points

The 20 marks in the "Mealtime behavior" category were used to reinforce sitting in his chair during the meal, requesting food rather than grabbing for it, and generally good meal behavior, such as using utensils properly and using a napkin. Purchase of snacks and the special meal for lunch and dinner could only be made with marks that D.L. had earned in his mealtime behavior category. The "Grown-up suggestions" category was used to reinforce compliance with staff requests. The plus points available for this category were given just as the mark were, but they did not figure into his regular economy. Plus points could be accumulated toward a "special deal," which was a special activity with his Intramural Counselor. Marks in the "General" category were used to reinforce appropriate interactions, particularly those with peers. The plus points accumulated in this category were also saved for "special deals."

Minimum appropriate behaviors. Since D.L. had exhibited a deficiency in the performance of the routine self-care behaviors, a number of these were reinforced with marks. Additional control over his behaviors was sought by restricting the spending of these marks to certain powerful backups. In order to eat the special meal at breakfast, D.L. was required to be out of bed on time, make his bed, dress neatly, have his room neat, and have his closets and drawers neat. In order for D.L. to have a bedtime story read to him, he was required to take a shower, put out his lanudry, and be in his room at bedtime. Since his proficiency at many of these behaviors was initially so low, the criterion for receiving a mark for behaviors, such as making his bed or being dressed neatly, was quite low to begin with. However, as he became more proficient, more was expected of him in order to receive a mark.

School. D.L. was not initially placed in group classes in the school program. During this period, his school program consisted of one-to-one sessions. He was able to earn 10 spendable marks for his performance during these sessions.

Punishment. D.L. was initially assigned to the time-out punishment condition. He remained on this condition throughout his Level I program.

Special procedures. D.L. was not allowed to spend marks saved from one day to the next for anything other than store. Thus, most reinforcing activities were not available to him unless he was earning marks. Plus points were used with D.L. to make additional marks available, but they were in the form of a bonus that did not figure into the regular economy. These plus points were given in the same way marks were; however, they were not spent in the regular manner, but they were saved for a special activity with his Intramural Counselor.

Length of program. D.L. remained on this program for eight weeks before beginning his Level II program.

Level II

Appropriate social behaviors. Reinforcement for mealtime behavior was discontinued on this program, but two additional categories of social behaviors were identified as targets, making a total of four targets. These targets were labeled as follows:

>Interaction — 15 marks + plus points
>Playing by yourself — 10 marks + plus points
>Grownup suggestions — 5 marks + plus points
>General — 10 marks + plus points

Marks in the "Interaction" category were used to reinforce any appropriate interactions between D.L. and other children. Staff was to be particularly sensitive to giving these marks if D.L. was playing with the younger children or was interacting appropriately in a group setting. The "Playing by yourself" category was used to reinforce D.L. whenever he was engaged in some appropriate, solitary activity. Marks in this category were not to be given, if he was playing by himself, when it was possible for him to be playing with other children. Marks in the "General" category continued to be given for any appropriate behavior, but emphasis was placed on those situations where D.L. performed an appropriate behavior, such as putting away a toy without a staff prompt being necessary. The "Grownup suggestions" category continued to be used to reinforce compliance with staff requests.

Minimum appropriate behaviors. The same procedures used on Level I were also used on this program to reinforce self-care behaviors. These procedures were changed, however, twelve weeks after D.L. began his Level II program. The same behaviors continued to be reinforced, but the procedures used were altered. In order for D.L. to earn a special meal at breakfast, both he and his roommate were required to have made their beds, picked up the room, straightened their closets and drawers, and to be neatly dressed. Also, for D.L. to stay up one-half hour later than the regular bedtime, both he and his roommate were required to take a shower, put out their laundry, and be in their room at bedtime. This procedure was set up not only to deal with the self-care behaviors but also, hopefully, to foster some concern and cooperation between D.L. and his roommate.

School. At this point, D.L. was attending group classes in the school. His school program was set up so that he was receiving marks for such behaviors as working independently, being on task, listening, waiting his turn, and getting started. He was able to earn a total of 20 spendable marks for these behaviors.

Punishment. Six weeks after beginning this program, all punishment procedures were removed for a four-week period. After this four weeks of no punishment contingencies, the response-cost procedures were started.

Length of program. D.L. remained on this program for twenty weeks before beginning Level II-Phase II.

Level II — Phase II

Appropriate social behaviors. Five categories of social behavior were identified as targets on this program. These targets were as follows:

Individual Programs

Accepting decisions — 10 marks + plus points
Interaction — 15 marks + plus points
Helping and sharing — 5 marks + plus points
Saying nice things — 5 marks + plus points
General — 10 marks + plus points

Marks in the "Accepting decisions" category were used to reinforce D.L. whenever he complied with a staff suggestion quickly and with a positive attitude. The 15 marks in the "Interaction" category were used to reinforce good interactions, especially those that occurred with the younger children or in a group setting. Staff was instructed to be particularly alert and to reinforce D.L. for handling situations in which another child was annoying or provoking him. Marks in the "Helping and sharing" category were used to reinforce any incidents of helping or sharing, especially if they occurred with the younger children. The "Saying nice things" category was used to reinforce any positive statements about or to other children. The 10 marks in the "General" category were used to reinforce any appropriate behavior, especially those that had been emphasized in earlier programs, such as appropriate meal behavior and playing by himself.

Minimum appropriate behaviors. At this point in his program, D.L. no longer had a roommate so that the procedures used on Level II to reinforce self-care behaviors were no longer used on this program. D.L. earned the special breakfast by making his bed, having his room neat, straightening his closets and drawers, and being dressed neatly. In order to stay up one-half hour later than the regular bedtime, he was required to shower, put out his laundry, and be in his room at bedtime.

School. D.L. continued to earn 20 spendable marks for good behavior in school. These marks were given for the same kinds of behaviors as listed on Level II.

Punishment. D.L. remained on the response-cost punishment condition for the first ten weeks of this program. At that point, D.L. was returned to time-out punishment.

Special procedures. A special procedure was developed with D.L. that enabled him to earn special staff attention. Three squares were designated on his mark sheet as "reward boxes." These boxes were the fifteenth box in the "Interaction" category, the fifth in the "Helping and sharing" category, and the fifth box in "Saying nice things." When D.L. earned a mark in one of these special boxes, he was entitled to five minutes alone with a staff member. D.L. was allowed to accumulate these five-minute periods, and they could be spent just talking with a staff member, going for a walk, or going to the Adler cafeteria with a staff member for a coke.

Length of program. At the end of the research project, D.L. was still in the treatment program and had been on this program for eleven weeks.

Home Program

D.L.'s home visits were not as frequent, or as routine, as those of many of the children in the program. Initially, it was felt that regular home visits would be more beneficial if they came after D.L. had made some gains in the cottage program and after some work had been done with the family. A student social worker was assigned to work with D.L.'s parents to teach them the basic principles of behavior modification and to set up procedures that they could use with D.L. when he was home. The parents responded well to this program and were able to implement some more consistent ways of dealing with D.L. during his home visits. Transportation difficulties somewhat restricted the frequency of home visits. Each time that D.L. made a home visit, the train schedules were such that his mother had to spend several hours on the cottage. This gave her a chance to observe D.L. in the cottage program and also allowed cottage staff an opportunity to discuss D.L.'s home visit with her. Two of the home visits also included spending half days in the classroom that he will be entering when he leaves Adler. The public-school teacher also made visits to observe him in the Adler classroom. The social worker at D.L.'s prospective school kept up with D.L.'s Adler program and began working with the family to coordinate the home program with the cottage program.

Data

Independent Observations

Cottage. The observers' ratings of D.L.'s interactions are of particular interest since interactions were reinforced in the "General" category during his Level I program and were identified as a target on his Level II program. After his Level I program began, there was some slight increase, but the rate was quite erratic, and there was no stable pattern of improvement. After his Level II program began, interaction was labeled as a target and there was some increase in the percentage of positive peer interaction. The percentage of peer interactions, which were rated positive during ten of the first thirteen weeks of the Level II program, showed an increase over the mean frequency observed during Orientation Level. After the Christmas break, the percentage of peer interactions that were positive seemed to stabilize at a higher rate and this gain was maintained for the rest of the Level II program. After Level II-Phase II began, the rate of positive peer interactions was fairly stable and at a frequency that showed a respectable gain over that observed during Orientation Level. There was, however, a slight decline during the last four weeks (Fig. 13).

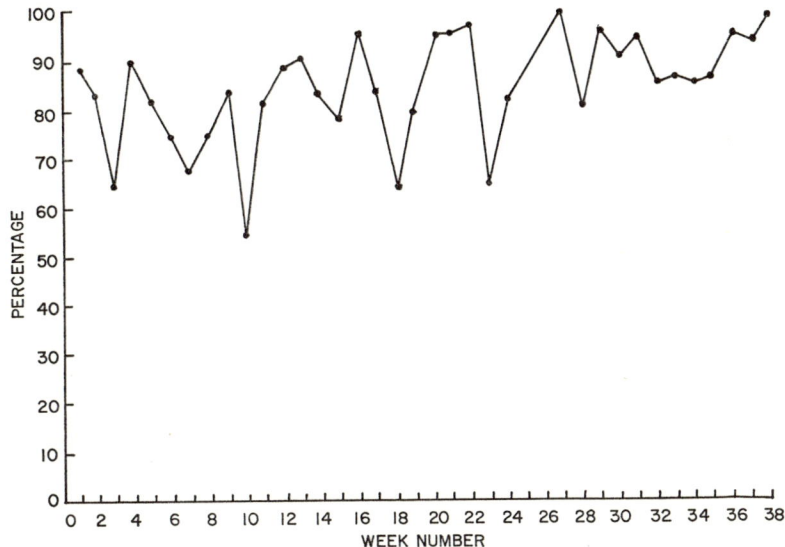

Figure 13. Subject 21, unit independent observations, percentage of positive peer interactions.

The percent of all D.L.'s interactions that were rated positive also indicated some gains. These gains were most evident and more stable after the Christmas break.

The percentage of time that D.L. was observed to be engaged in a positive, solitary activity is of some interest since a category labeled "Playing by yourself" was a target when D.L.'s Level II program began. Some gain was made in this category after the Level I program began, even though it wasn't identified as a target. After his Level II program began, there was some fluctuation, although the observed rate was generally higher than it was during Orientation Level. "Playing by yourself" ceased to be a target on Level II-Phase II, but the percent of time engaged in a positive, solitary activity continued at a high rate for eight weeks. The last four weeks showed a more erratic pattern with a downward trend (Fig. 14).

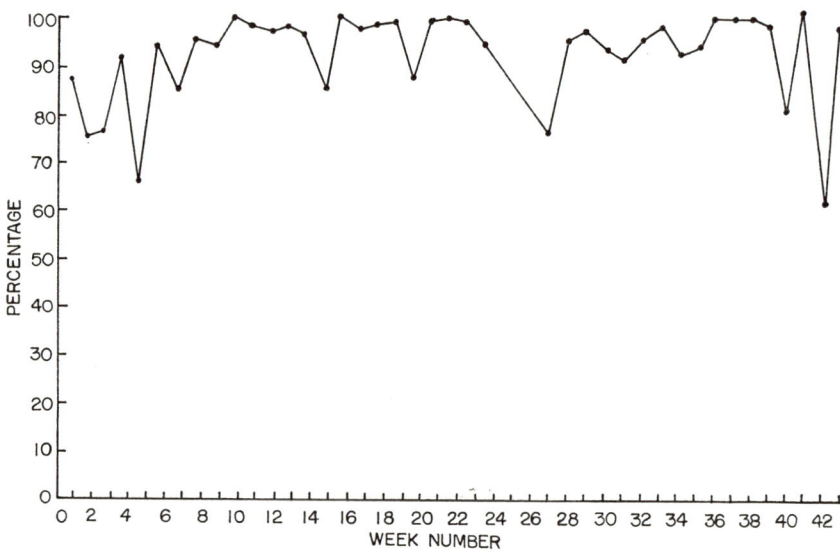

Figure 14. Subject 21, unit independent observations, percentage of time engaged in solitary activities.

The percentage of verbalizations which were observed to be positive is of interest, since "Saying nice things" was identified as a target during Level II-Phase II. The data does not indicate any particular change as a result of tokening positive verbalizations during Level II-Phase II. Overall, however, there did appear to be some gain made in the percentage of verbalizations that were positive over the percentage that was observed during Orientation Level.

School. D.L. attended school only one week, while he was on Orientation Level. After his program began, there was an immediate decrease in deviant behavior over the 16 percent that was observed during Orientation Level. This gain was maintained until week 28, and since that time, the pattern is more erratic with some weeks showing considerable incidences of deviant behavior.

Individual Programs

The percentage of all D.L.'s interactions which were observed to be positive showed an increase when his Level I program began over the rate that was observed during the week he was on Orientation Level. The percentage of his classroom interactions which were judged positive was generally quite high until week 31, when a more variable and somewhat lower pattern began to emerge.

Daily Checklist

Those behaviors that were not felt to require systematic contingencies showed a considerable increase when the Level I program began. The percent performance of these behaviors was somewhat erratic, but this initial gain was generally maintained throughout the rest of D.L.'s program.

Appropriate meal behavior was identified as a target on D.L.'s Level I program. During Orientation Level, D.L.'s performance of appropriate meal behavior was at a very low rate. After his Level I program began, there was an immediate increase in his performance. Gains made on Level I were maintained, even after marks were not given on his Level II program (Fig. 15). A number of items on the Daily Checklist resulted in special contingencies. Making his bed,

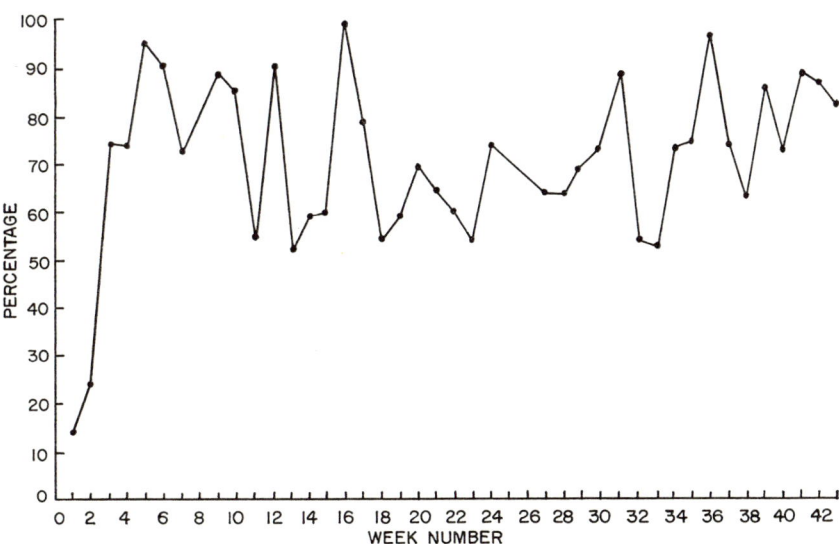

Figure 15. Subject 21, performance of minimum appropriate behaviors—meal behavior.

dressing neatly, having his room neat, and having his closets and drawers neat resulted in both marks and a Premack of the special breakfast. Putting out his laundry and taking a shower also resulted in marks and a Premack of a bedtime story. D.L.'s performance of these behaviors generally increased after his Level I program started. Midway in his Level II program, the program was revised and the contingencies used with these behaviors were altered. No marks were used, just Premack contingencies and the additional constraint in which his roommate was required to perform the same behaviors in order for both of them to receive the Premack contingency. His performance of these behaviors remained approximately the same on this program. However, there seemed to be less variability. When Level II-Phase II began, D.L. no longer had a roommate and the Premack contingency applied just to D.L. On this program, the rate of performance of these behaviors showed an increase, and during the last three weeks, his rate of performance was nearly perfect (Fig. 16).

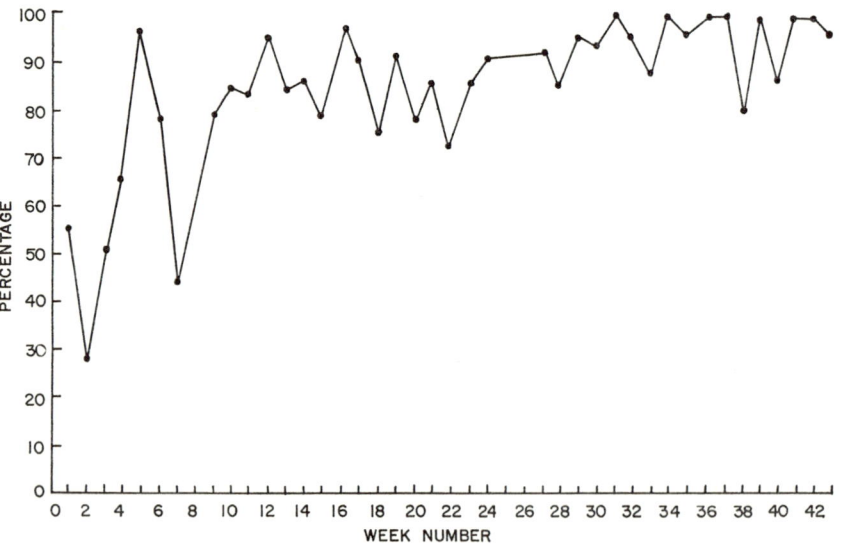

Figure 16. Subject 21, performance of minimum appropriate behaviors—bed made, room neat, closets and drawers neat, dressed neatly, shower, laundry.

Punishment Data

During Orientation Level, D.L. exhibited a very high frequency (average of 46 per day) of those behaviors defined as punishable.

The most frequent category of punishable behavior was defiance, with an average of 31 incidents per day. D.L. also exhibited a relatively high frequency of those behaviors labeled "minor assault," i.e. shoving, pushing, pinching.

Institution of the time-out procedures brought the average frequency of punishable behavior down to two and a half per day. This decrease occurred almost immediately and was maintained throughout the time-out condition. Before the response-cost procedures were instituted, all punishment conditions were suspended for a two-week period. During this time, there was only a slight increase in the frequency of punishable behaviors over that observed during the time-out condition. It is not surprising that the frequency of punishable behavior was much lower during this second baseline period than it was during the initial baseline, since a positive program that reinforced incompatible behaviors was in effect during this second baseline (Fig. 17).

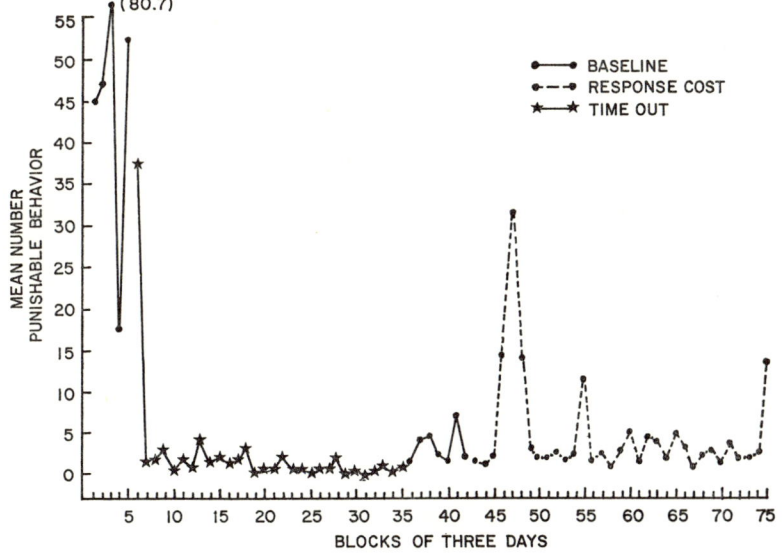

Figure 17. Subject 21, frequency of punishable behavior.

When response cost was begun, the relatively low level of punishable behavior that was observed during the baseline period was maintained. After a short time, however, there was considerable acceleration in the frequency of punishable behavior. This acceleration lasted for nine days before the frequency of punishable behavior was again reduced to the rate observed before. This lower rate was maintained for approximately two weeks, and from that point forward, a more variable pattern emerged. Over the entire response-cost condition, D.L. averaged five and one-half incidents per day, which was higher than the three and one-half incidents per day observed during the second baseline period. Thus, while the rate of punishable behavior during response cost was lower than that observed during the initial baseline, it was not lower than the rate observed during the second baseline. Thus, it would seem that response cost tended to have an eliciting rather than a suppressing effect on D.L.'s frequency of punishable behavior (Fig. 17).

Chapter 8

PUNISHMENT STUDY

WITHIN the context of the milieu (Chapter 2), a study was conducted to investigate the effects of response-cost and time-out punishment procedures on undesirable behavior. The list of punishable behaviors (Dimension 5) used in this study was developed between February, 1968, and February, 1969. The study was begun in February, 1969, and continued until May, 1970. Eighteen children were included in the study.

Upon admission to the cottage, children were assigned randomly to one of two conditions, time out or response cost. During Orientation Level, the frequency of punishable behavior was recorded by staff, but no systematic consequences were applied to these behaviors. This period of two to three weeks provided a baseline, which served as a reference point in evaluating the effects of both punishment procedures. At the end of Orientation Level, the punishment procedures were instituted as a consequence of those behaviors that were defined as punishable. The child received the form of punishment that was dictated by the random assignment, until it appeared that some stable effect was evidenced. At this point, the child was shifted to the other punishment condition. Thus, each child in the study received both forms of punishment, but the order in which they received the conditions was varied. Nine children received time out first, followed by response cost; nine received response cost first, followed by time out. During later stages of the study, all punishment contingencies were suspended for some of the children, for a two-week period before the second punishment condition was instituted.

The time-out procedure used was to remove the child from the ongoing situation and to place him in an isolation room for a certain length of time. This room was a tiled room, $3 \times 5 \times 10$

feet, with an overhead light covered by a screen, and with either a small Plexiglass window or a small peephole in the door.

When a child emitted a punishable behavior, he would be told that because he had done "X," he would have to go to time out for a certain length of time. If the punishable behavior did not cease or if he emitted other punishable behaviors before he got to time out, then the time to be served was increased by half.

Response cost took the form of fines that the child paid with his earned marks. Payment of a fine was required before marks could be spent for any other purpose. When a child emitted a punishable behavior while on response cost, he was told that because of behavior "X," he was fined a certain number of marks. If the punishable behavior did not cease or if other punishable behaviors occurred in the situation, the child was fined for the occurrence of each of these behaviors. For punishable behaviors that were continuous in nature, such as tantrums, swearing, and defiance, a 15-second interval was defined as a single occurrence, and fines were applied to each 15-second interval of such behavior. See Appendix C for a complete description of the procedures used in administering time out and response cost.

Punishable behaviors were labeled and grouped into five categories, which were then arranged hierarchially according to the severity of the behavior. Staff rankings were used to establish this hierarchy, and penalties were assigned to the various categories. A relatively minor penalty was assigned to those behaviors in the first (100 Level) category, and the most severe punishment was assigned to behaviors in the fifth (500 Level) category. Categories for punishable behavior are the same as those listed in Chapter 2, pages 21 and 22. Only the 100 through 500 Levels of punishable behavior were included in the study. The 600 Level behaviors were not included because contingencies were invoked for these behaviors during Orientation Level. Contingencies for the 700 Level were not specified for all children, but these were determined on an individual basis for each child.

Time-out penalties were assigned to the five categories. The 100 Level behaviors resulted in 10 minutes in time out; 200 Level behaviors, 20 minutes; 300 Level behaviors, 30 minutes; 400

Level behaviors, 40 minutes; and the 500 Level behaviors, 50 minutes.

The amount of the response cost attached to each level depended upon the earning power, in marks per day, of the child. If the earning power was between 1 and 50 marks per day, the fines were 1, 2, 4, 8, and 12 marks for the 100, 200, 300, 400, and 500 Levels, respectively; if the earning power was between 51 and 85 marks per day, the fines for the levels were 2, 4, 8, 16, and 24 marks; if the earning power was from 86 to 115 marks per day, the fines were 3, 6, 12, 24, and 36 marks; if the earning power was over 115 marks per day, the fines were 4, 8, 16, 32, and 48 marks.

Results

The results of these procedures can be evaluated three ways: in terms of the effects across all 18 subjects; in terms of the effects upon the two groups formed by the initial assignment of the two categories; and in terms of the effect upon the individual subjects.

Effect Across All Subjects

For purposes of this analysis, the data for all 18 subjects was grouped without regard for the order of the punishment condition (Fig. 18). When the data was grouped in this fashion and the mean frequency of punishable behavior observed across all subjects during the time-out condition was compared with the mean frequency for all subjects during the baseline condition, the reduction observed during time out (TO) proved to be significantly different (all differences reported as significant had t values which were significant at the .05 level) from the baseline. When the same comparison was made for the response-cost condition, the mean frequency during response cost (RC) also proved to be significantly lower than the baseline level.

When the effects of TO and RC are viewed in terms of the levels of punishable behaviors, it was found that both TO and RC significantly reduced the frequency of the 100, 300, and 500 Level behaviors (Fig. 19). Only TO produced a significant reduction in 200 Level behaviors, and neither condition produced

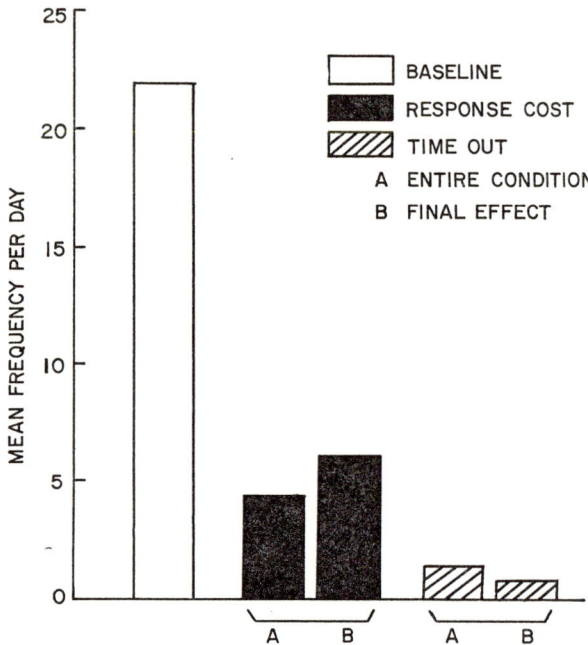

Figure 18. Mean frequency of punishable behavior across all subjects, N=18.

a significant reduction of 400 Level behaviors. This lack of effect on the 400 Level behaviors was undoubtedly due to the very low frequency of these behaviors during baseline.

A comparison was made between time out and response cost across all subjects, and the mean level of punishable behavior during the time-out condition was found to be significantly lower than the mean during the response-cost condition.

Since the length of time that a given subject spent on each condition depended upon the stabilization of his rate, there was considerable variation in the length of exposure to each condition across subjects. There was also some variation in the length of time that subjects spent on the baseline condition. In order to evaluate the results for more equivalent time periods across subjects and also to assess the ultimate effect of both procedures, the results of the last "X" number of days a subject was on each

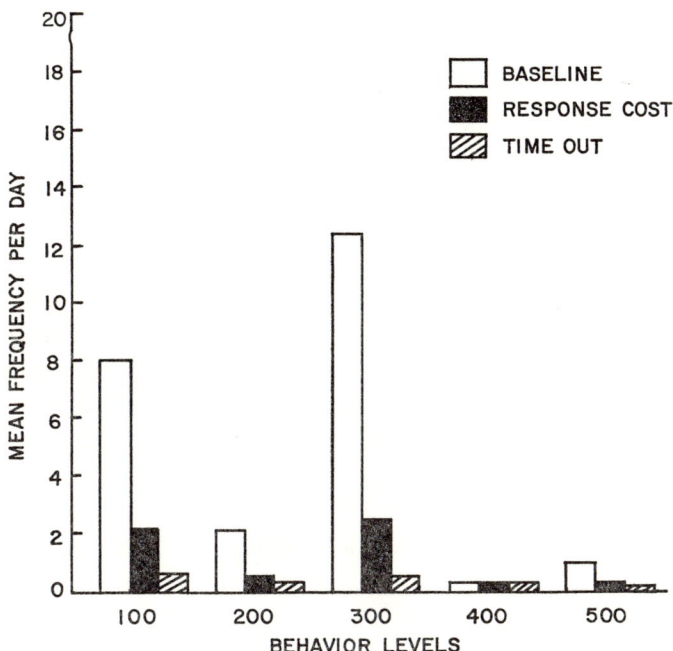

Figure 19. Mean frequency of the levels of punishable behaviors across all subjects, N=18.

condition was figured. The "X" number of days was determined by using the number each subject spent on baseline. This result, labeled "final effect," was figured for each subject for both the time-out and response-cost conditions. When the final effect of time out was grouped for all subjects and compared with the baseline, the final effect produced by time out was significantly lower than the baseline. The same result was found when the final effect of response cost was compared with the baseline. When the final effect of time out was compared with the final effect of response cost, the difference was not significant.

Differences Between the Two Groups

The initial random assignment of subjects to one of the two conditions produced two groups, each with nine subjects. One group (Subjects 12, 14, 15, 16, 18, 21, 24, 25, 26) received time out first and then response cost, while the other group (Subjects 9, 10, 13, 17, 19, 20, 23, 27, 28) received response cost first followed by time out. The comparisons reported in this section are concerned with these two groups.

While the baseline frequency of punishable behavior was higher for the group that received response cost first, it was not significantly higher. The two groups also did not differ significantly in the baseline frequency of any of the five levels of punishable behavior. Time out produced significant reductions in punishable behavior compared to the baseline, in both the group that received time out first and the group that received time out after response cost. Response cost also produced a significant reduction in punishable behavior compared to the baseline in both groups (Figs. 20 and 21).

When the effect of time out received first was compared to

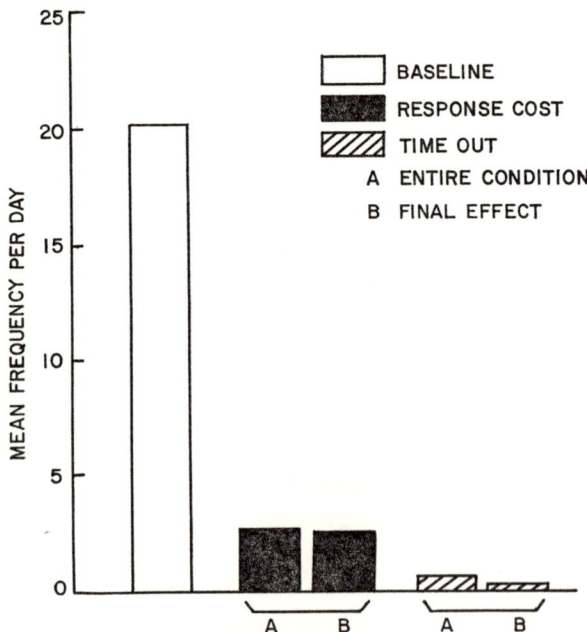

Figure 20. Mean frequency of punishable behavior for subjects receiving time out first and response cost second, N=19.

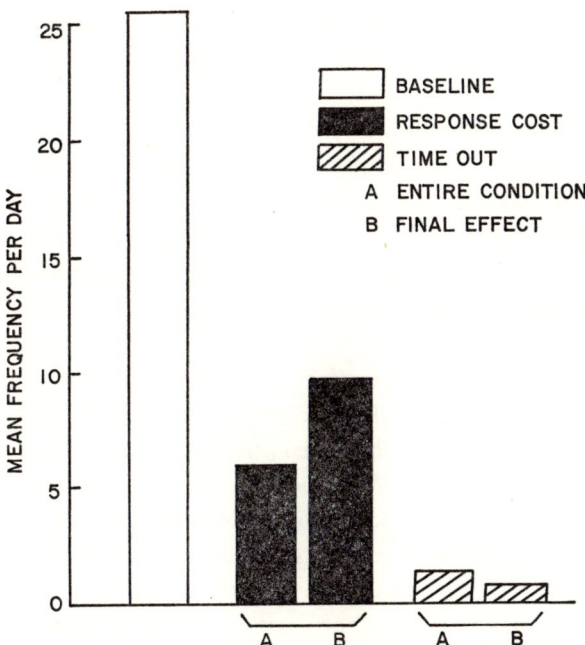

Figure 21. Mean frequency of punishable behavior for subjects receiving response cost first and time out second, N=19.

the effect of time out when it followed response cost, no significant difference was found. The same result was found when the effect of response cost first was compared with the effect of response cost after it followed time out. Thus, the effect of the punishment procedure was not significantly affected by the order in which it appeared.

Differences Within the Two Groups

When the effect of time out was compared with the effect of response cost in the group receiving time out first, no significant difference was found. No significant difference was found between response cost and time out when the same comparison was made in the group receiving response cost first (Figs. 20 and 21).

While the difference between the means of the response-cost and time-out conditions was much larger in the group that received response cost first, the variance in this group was also much larger and hence, the lack of a significant difference.

Effect Upon Individual Subjects

All subjects in the group receiving time out first showed a reduction in deviant behavior during both punishment conditions. Subject 21 showed a reduction during both conditions when compared to the initial baseline, although the response-cost condition did not reduce the rate over that observed during the second baseline.

The same result was true for the subjects in the group receiving response cost first with one exception. Subject 17 showed a higher rate on both punishment conditions than during Orientation Level. For Subject 17, response cost produced an extremely accelerated rate of punishable behavior. Institution of the time-out condition produced an immediate reduction, and after the first few days on time out, the rate of punishable behavior was reduced to approximately that observed during baseline.

For 15 of the 18 subjects, the mean rate of punishable behavior during the time-out condition was less than it was during the response-cost condition. Subjects 12, 13, and 27 were the exceptions. The mean rates for only Subject 25 were identical for both time out and response cost.

All punishment contingencies were discontinued for a two-week period, following the first punishment condition for four subjects in each group. For six of these eight subjects, the mean rate during this period, while higher than the rate during the punishment condition that preceded it, was lower than the rate observed during Orientation Level. For the other two subjects, the mean rate of punishable behavior, during this two-week period of no contingencies, was higher than the rate observed during Orientation Level.

For all but one (Subject 21) of these eight subjects, the reinstitution of a punishment contingency caused a decrease in the rate of punishable behavior observed while no contingencies were in effect.

Discussion

In evaluating the results, it must be kept in mind that this study was not conducted in a laboratory setting where all variables, other than the one being manipulated, were controlled. This study was conducted within an ongoing service program where a great many uncontrolled and possibly confounding influences were operating.

During Orientation Level, the 100 through 500 Level punishment contingencies were not in effect. Nevertheless, certain influences were operating that might conceivably have had some bearing on the rate and pattern of punishable behavior observed during this period. One was the drastic change in environment that the child experienced when he began residential treatment. This frequently operated to suppress undesirable behavior initially and created the phenomenon referred to as the "honeymoon period." The honeymoon period was typically followed by an increase in undesirable behavior. While this phenomenon was observed with many of the children in this study, it did not occur with all of them. Some children responded to this new situation by showing a high frequency of undesirable behavior initially and a lower frequency as the situation became more familiar and other influences exerted themselves. Another possible influence during Orientation Level was the fact that children entering the program had the opportunity to observe the consequences that other children experienced as a result of certain behaviors. They thus learned the rules and requirements of the program before they actually experienced any contingencies themselves. This exposure to the behavior of other children did not always operate to reduce undesirable behavior. Some children showed signs of learning new forms of undesirable behavior from observing other children on the unit.

In addition, reinforcers were available to the child noncontingently during Orientation Level. Consequently, the feedback system (Dimension 4) was inadequate at this time, because the expected appropriate behaviors (Dimensions 2, 3) and the punishable behaviors had not been made explicit to the child.

Since there were many physical and social variables interacting with each other in the milieu program, there was no direct way of assessing whether or not the changes in the frequency of punishable behavior were due to the use of punishment contingencies. Indirect evidence did indicate that the reductions observed were probably not due to other aspects of the program alone. The fact that two different punishment procedures were used with each individual with somewhat different results, while the other aspects of the program were in operation with both procedures, suggested that the punishment system was having some effect. The removal of all punishment contingencies for eight subjects, while the other aspects of the program continued to operate, also gave some evidence that the suppression effect that was observed was not totally due to the programming and reinforcing of incompatible responses.

But the question of whether other parts of the program or punishment procedures produced the greater change in the frequency of punishable behavior was not the question of interest in this study. This study's purpose was to evaluate the relative effects of two punishment procedures when used within a treatment milieu.

Besides the confoundedness of the punishment and the other dimensions of the milieu, there were many variables operating in the situation that conceivably could have influenced the frequency of punishable behavior, such as getting a new roommate, a favorite staff member leaving, visits by the parents, no visits by the parents, teasing by other children, and so on ad infinitum. While influences such as these may have affected the pattern or rate of change evidenced by a single child, it does seem reasonable to assume that variables such as these were not operating in any systematic way across subjects. It also seems reasonable to assume that uncontrolled variables of this type would be operating in any applied setting; and the focus of the study was whether or not, given a fluid situation such as this, these procedures would have any impact. The fact that there appears to be a fair amount of consistency in the results across subjects suggests that the procedures being used did exert a considerable amount of influence.

Certain problems were encountered in connection with the implementation of both punishment procedures. With time out, a procedure evolved whereby a child was allowed a reasonable length of time to go voluntarily to time out before physical force was used. A child was prompted that he would have to serve "X" time for "X" offenses and that the time to be served would be increased by half if he did not go immediately. If he did not go, he was told that he could not participate in any activity until his time was served. Then he was ignored until he made some indication that he was ready to serve his time. If he became actively belligerent or continued to misbehave, then he was taken physically to the time-out room. This procedure seemed to work surprisingly well, especially for the older children.

The response-cost procedure was set up so that if a child owed more in fines than he had earned, he was in debt and was not allowed to spend marks for anything until he was out of debt. The procedure generated problems since some children, especially the younger ones, became deeply entrenched in debt. Some were in debt to the extent that they would have had to work for weeks before they could possibly pay off the fines. This meant that they had to perform for long periods of time with little tangible payoff. Faced with this prospect, some children developed a "what have I got to lose" attitude, which undoubtedly generated more punishable behavior. No one procedure was established to deal with this problem. When it occured with an individual child, a procedure was worked out to enable him to work his way out of debt more rapidly. One procedure used was to match the number of marks paid toward his fine by some factor. i.e. if the child paid 10 marks, 50 might actually be subtracted from the total. This procedure was used with younger children without their becoming aware that they were not paying off the entire fine themselves. This deception was possible because of their lack of number concepts. With the older children, two different kinds of procedures were used. One involved giving bonus marks for especially good performances, e.g. earning all marks in a target area or not receiving additional fines. The other procedure involved making available certain of the reinforcers on a daily basis, even though the fine was not paid off, contingent upon not receiving any further fines. All these special procedures for handling fines were felt to be successful. It is conceivable that the response-cost results for some of the subjects might have taken a different form if these procedures had been adopted earlier.

One cannot make truly comparative statements about the results of two totally disparate procedures, since there is no way they can be equated on a number of parameters that might affect their relative outcomes. With punishment procedures, intensity is a critical factor and is one that can be expected to influence the results of each procedure. There is no way of knowing whether the two procedures used in this study were indeed equal in intensity. Thus, comparative statements about time out and response cost can only be given to the specific procedures used in this study. The fact that time out was found to have the greater impact across subjects may not have been the case if different response-cost values had been used. A great deal of research in this area is needed before any generalizations regarding the relative effects of time out and response cost can be made.

Summary

Eighteen subjects received both time-out and response-cost punishment procedures. Nine received time out first and nine received response cost first. Significant reductions were observed with both procedures. Across all subjects, time out produced significantly more reduction than response cost. This difference between time out and response cost was not found when the data for the two groups was analyzed. No significant differences were found in relation to the order in which the conditions were assigned. Only one subject showed no reduction in punishable behavior with either condition. One other subject evidenced reduction with response cost in comparison to the initial baseline on Orientation Level, but not in relation to a second baseline between punishment conditions. All other subjects evidenced reduction with both conditions.

In general, it can be said that the time-out procedures used in this study were more effective than the response-cost procedures.

Chapter 9

ASSESSMENT OF THE RESEARCH PROJECT

THIS RESEARCH project has been described as a process study in which the major goal was conceptualizing an ongoing service program in such a manner that the crucial, therapeutic variables could be identified, taught, replicated, and evaluated (Chapter 1). Thus, the conceptualization of the milieu (interrelated, independent variables) was the first major step in the process. Chapter 2 has presented the conceptualization of the milieu.

Assessment of the Conceptualization and Implementation

The following is a summary of the level of development and function of each dimension of the milieu at the end of the research project.

Dimension 1

Dimension 1, a progressive movement system, served as the program anchor. The Orientation Level served as a period of observation and planning, the three treatment levels clearly focused on the goal of the treatment program, i.e. returning the child to the community. While the treatment levels, as stated, served as clear guidelines for program development, achieving all levels was not necessary before a child was allowed to return to the community. In some cases, it was possible to continue his program development after returning to the community. Thus, the rate and level of movement were not the criterion measure of the child's progress. This dimension, however, served as a guideline for measuring progress as well as for program planning.

Dimension 2

Dimension 2, daily routines and minimum appropriate self-care behaviors, served several purposes:

1. The itemized list of minimum appropriate behaviors (MAB) which constituted the Daily Checklist was the research instrument that served to record whether or not the child's routine self-care behaviors were performed. Data was collected also on this instrument during Orientation Level;

2. The record of the child's performance on Orientation Level served as a guideline for developing his treatment program;

3. Daily routine activities on the cottage were structured around the Daily Checklist, and thus the check list served as a training instrument for allocating staff time and activities;

4. Achievement of the MAB targets served as a meausre of the child's progress.

Dimension 3

Dimension 3, appropriate social behaviors, served as a guideline for developing the treatment targets for each child. While this was one of the most important dimensions, it was not as well conceptualized as was needed. The following developmental steps are recommended:

1. Four of the six categories of appropriate social behavior, i.e. cooperative behavior, participation, interaction, and constructive, should be further conceptualized in a manner that would allow them to be operationalized in terms of appropriate social task to be performed. The categories, helping and sharing, should be incorporated into the cooperation category.

2. The content of the milieu program should be structured to offer the opportunity for each of these tasks to be performed.

3. A measure of the performance should be made at the Orientation Level as was done with Dimension 2 (MAB). Thus, this measure of appropriate social behaviors could serve as a more useful guideline in developing the treatment targets. In addition, the instrument should be developed to measure the movement of the child in the increase of prosocial behaviors, e.g. in a manner similar to the measure of decrease in punishable behaviors in Dimension 5. The appropriate social behaviors should be plugged into the independent observations in the same way that the punishable behaviors were.

These suggested developments would serve to increase the amount of focus placed on increasing prosocial behaviors, make the content of the milieu program more specific, enhance the staff training, improve the individual programming, improve the measures of change.

Dimension 4

Dimension 4, a system of feedback and reinforcement, served as a major communication system in the cottage. It communicated the program target goals for each child and the daily progress toward these goals. It was a means of communicating approval and rewarding appropriate behavior. Initially, this dimension was used as a measure of progress (token earning); this was recognized as an inappropriate measure of progress.

Additional ways of communicating with the child were tried experimentally on the project and would seem to warrant further development. The first of these techniques would be role-playing situations in which the child could be taught in advance to relate to an anticipated situation. Thus, when he encountered the situation, he would have the skills at his command, e.g. teaching the child to wait his turn in a public-school situation before he entered the public school. This approach would recognize the child's capacity to anticipate and plan for events. Another role-playing situation would be for a staff member to model an example of the child's punishable behavior and to let the child state what contingency would be invoked for that behavior. This situation could help the child to see the relation between his behavior and the consequences.

A second technique would be to use video tape. For example, the staff could tape the child's behavior in a given situation and allow him to see the tape; then staff could discuss his behavior with him. This technique could be used to demonstrate both prosocial and punishable behaviors.

Thus, it is suggested that the continued development of this dimension would emphasize an input-feedback system, with increased emphasis on the cognitive process involved in changing behavior.

Dimension 5

Dimension 5, the punishment system, conceptualized and operationalized a set of punishable behaviors appropriate to the milieu. The method used to develop this set of behaviors appears to be applicable to other settings as are most of the specific behaviors identified in the milieu. A systematic set of contingencies were outlined, i.e. amount of time out and/or response cost. These two conditions, time out and response cost, were studied (Chapter 8).

Other Aspects of the Project

One major aspect of the conceptualization of project phenomena was the orientation to the child in the milieu. Chapter 3 has made the major aspects of this orientation explicit. However, some aspects of this orientation might be stated in such a manner that they could be taught more effectively and that their existence could be measured with regard to the direct care staff.

Another major aspect of the project was the development of instruments for ongoing evaluation of the child's change in the milieu and his continued change after his return to the community. The development of these instruments has been described in Chapter 4. The two most important deficits in the instrument development were discussed in relation to development of Dimension 3. These deficits were the need for a more adequate instrument for measuring change in prosocial behaviors and for greater precision in measures of prosocial behavior in the instrument used by independent observers.

An additional aspect of the conceptualization of the project was the continued implementation of the child's program in his home and community, i.e. the concept of continuity of care. This is discussed in Dimension 1. Many channels were opened up for this aspect of the project to develop and, in varying degrees, continuity of care was achieved for many of the children (Chapters 6 and 7). Research money and, in turn, research time made it impractical to develop this aspect of the program as fully as was desired. In addition, it is hypothesized that a more adequate development of Dimension 3 would facilitate the development of home and community programs.

Assessment of Outcome

The ultimate evaluation of the research project is the evidence of durable, prosocial change in the children who were served in the project. It is convenient to assess outcome in two ways.

In comparative studies, measures are made of the differences between the effects of one set of interventions (independent variables) as compared to another set, and/or between the set of interventions used in this project as compared to a control group in which no interventions were used. As stated earlier, it was not possible to implement a comparative study until an adequate conceptualization of the project procedure was achieved. The main purpose of this study was to conceptualize the process. In follow-up studies, a comparison is made for each child in relation to the change that occurred in his functioning before admission to the project and following discharge. Even though the period of time between the close of the project and the writing of this manuscript has been short, a pilot follow-up study was completed on those children who had been discharged long enough for any evaluation. It is recognized that this study, as follows, is a very preliminary step in the development of an adequate outcome-assessment procedure.

Pilot Follow-up Study

The items of the follow-up questionnaires were derived from the pool of behavior problems that were found to be common to children admitted to the research project program at Cottage G. The typical item provided a brief statement of some behavior and asked for an estimate of the frequency of the behavior and an opinion about whether or not his behavior was a problem (Appendix G, Parent Questionnaire and School Questionnaire).

The primary objective of the questionnaires was to record from persons in the home and school setting, parents or guardians and classroom teachers, their current perceptions of the status of behavior problems of the child. Whenever it was possible, some perception of the amount or lack of behavioral change was elicited, i.e. when the person interviewed had lived and/or worked with the child prior to admission and after discharge.

The questionnaires were administered in the style of a structured interview in order to increase the chances for complete and accurate data. The interview procedure allowed a trained person from the research staff to present the questions orally, rephrasing for clarification if necessary, and to record all of the data. Oral presentation allowed the interviewer to elicit estimates of behavior frequency and perceptions of problems. This was necessary because many of the parents/guardians of the children had difficulty reading, writing, and dealing with such tasks as filling out questionnaires. In the process of developing the questionnaires, the items and the interviewing procedure were tested by different interviewers on parents who were participating in child-management classes.

The questionnaires were administered by the Project Coordinator, Extramural Case Coordinators, and research assistants, depending upon who could be in the right place at the right time. In a few cases, the questionnaires had to be left for teachers and parents to fill out independently.

Description of the Sample

Of the 30 children whose data have been used for this report, seven were still residing at the cottage when the collection of follow-up data was initiated and completed.

Of the 23 children who had been discharged, five children were not included in the follow-up investigation. Three children were discharged too recently for any meaningful follow-up activity to be undertaken. One child spent a little less than three months at the cottage before she was taken from the cottage by her parents. The staff felt that she had not been in the program long enough for any significant changes to have occurred, and it was felt that any follow-up data obtained would be hard to interpret. The fifth child was taken from the cottage by her family because of decisions they had made about future medical treatment for her. She was not included in the sample because the physical health problems of this child presented insurmountable complications for interpreting any follow-up data.

Thus, there were 18 children for which follow-up data was sought. The sample included 13 boys and 5 girls, whose age at the follow-up interviews ranged from 8 years, 5 months to 15 years, 1 month with an average of 12 years, 5 months. On the average, the interval between the discharge date and follow-up interview was 8.8 months with a range of 2 to 16 months. Average length of residence was 8.3 months with a range of 3 to 12 months. School data was obtained on all 18 children, but data from the parents or guardian was obtainable for only 16.

Analyses of the Data

Before the data from the follow-up questionnaire was organized, data from the preadmission reports for each child was summarized with respect to the following:
1. Problems in the family with the parents and siblings.
2. Personal problems.
3. School problems with the teacher, peer group, or academic Achievement.
4. Neighborhood problems with adults and children.
5. Previous contacts with agencies for adjustment problems.

Two summaries of the problems listed on the follow-up questionnaires were prepared, one each for data from home and data from school. These problems listed on follow-up summaries were compared with preadmission problem summaries and each problem for each child was classified as follows:
1. Present problem was listed in preadmission report.
2. Present problem was not listed in preadmission report.

Four research assistants, who were graduate students in clinical psychology with no previous exposure to the children, served as raters for the research project. These raters were given summaries of preadmission problems, follow-up data, and a Follow-up Rating Form (Appendix G) that was devised to classify the children and their problems.

There were four categories for classifying present problems

that were listed as preadmission problems. A present problem could be rated as follows:

1. More serious than prior to admission.
2. Much like problem prior to admission—improvement questionable.
3. Still existing but less serious than prior to admission.
4. Not different than would be expected of a normal child.

After all the ratings were made, averages of judges' ratings across the four categories were taken (Table III). In addition, ratings of each child's problems in two adjustment areas, home and school, were averaged to give an overall score for the child in each of the categories.

The data showed that those problems classified as home were rated 55 percent as improved, and 27 percent as improved to a degree that they were considered indistinguishable from problems of normal children. One out of the 33 problems under home designation was rated as more serious than prior to admission. Five problems under home designation, 15 percent of the total, were classified as improvement questionable.

For those problems occurring in the school setting (Table III), 53 percent, 28 of a total of 53, were classified as improved; and 7 percent were rated improved to a degree that they were considered indistinguishable from the problems of normal children. Twenty-one problems, 40 percent, rated in the questionable improvement category. No problems in the school setting were rated as more serious than prior to admission.

TABLE III
RATING OF CHILD'S BEHAVIOR AT FOLLOW-UP COMPARED TO PREADMISSION

Rating Intervals	Rating Categoriees	Children				Problems			
		Home Number Children	%	School Number Problems	%	Home Number Children	%	School Number Problems	%
4.00	Normal	2	14			9	27	4	7
3.00–3.99	Improved	9	65	10	56	18	55	28	53
2.00–2.99	Improvement questionable	2	14	8	44	5	15	21	40
1.00–1.99	Worse	1	7			1	3		
	Totals	14	100	18	100	33	100	53	100

When the ratings of the children's home and school problems were averaged to give a composite score for each child's home and school problems, the results in Table III were obtained.

Two children (Subjects 8 and 18), or 14 percent, were rated as functioning as normals in the home setting. Nine children (Subjects 1, 6, 7, 11, 13, 15, 19, 20, and 22), or 65 percent, were rated as improved in the home setting. Two children (Subjects 5 and 9), 14 percent, fell in the questionable improvement range; and one child (Subject 14), 7 percent, was rated unimproved.

Within the school setting, 10 children (Subjects 4, 7, 8, 10, 11, 13, 15, 19, 20, and 22), or 56 percent, were rated improved. Eight children (Subjects, 1, 2, 3, 5, 6, 9, 14, and 18), or 44 percent, had averages that fell in the questionable improvement range.

The present problems that were different from those prior to admission were classified by the kind of professional intervention that the rater felt would be appropriate. The raters were asked to choose between the following five alternatives:

1. Residential treatment.
2. Long-term outpatient services of 10 or more weekly sessions.
3. Short-term outpatient services of 5 to 10 weekly sessions.
4. Limited consultation with parents and/or teachers.
5. No professional intervention.

With respect to present problems different from the presenting problems, four children (Subjects 2, 5, 9, and 19) were classified as needing outpatient services of a long-term nature, i.e. 10 or more weekly sessions; 11 children (Subjects 1, 3, 6, 8, 10, 11, 13, 14, 15, 20, and 22) were classified as needing short-term outpatient services, i.e. five to ten weekly sessions; two children (Subjects 7 and 18) were classified as cases that needed limited consultative services with parents or teachers. Ratings were not obtained for this question for one child who had no additional problems listed (Subject 4).

Summary

In summary, 18 of the 30 cottage children were followed up. Thirteen of these children were boys; and on an average, the length of residence for the group was 8.3 months. At the time of the follow-up interview, the average age of the group was 12 years, 5 months; and the interval, between discharge and the follow-up interview, averaged 8.8 months.

Data was obtained from the school personnel for all 18 children, but data from the families was obtained for only 14 of the 18 cases. This data, summarized and rated, revealed that people in the home setting reported that 82 percent of the problems had improved. The data from the school setting revealed that 60 percent of the problems had improved, 23 percent had not improved, and improvement was questionable for the remaining 17 percent. Within the home setting, 79 percent of the children were rated improved or better.

Thirty-seven percent of the children had present problems that the raters felt merited the attention of professionals on a short-term, outpatient basis. Ten percent of the children were seen as needing long-term out-patient services. Six percent of the children needed limited consultative services with parents or teachers. None were recommended for residential care.

REFERENCES

Ayllon, T., and Azrin, N.: *The Token Economy: A Motivational System for Therapy and Rehabilitation.* New York, Appleton-Century-Crofts, 1968.

Bandura, A., and Walters, R.: *Social Learning and Personality Development.* New York, Holt, Rinehart & Winston, 1963.

Connaway, R. S.: *A Conceptual Formulation and Observational Scheme for Analysis of Social Work Practice: A Representation of the Object, Action, and Operating Principle in Social Work Practice,* Doctoral dissertation. Washington University, Ann Arbor, Michigan, University Microfilms, 1964, No. 65-6836.

Crane, J. A.: Utilizing the fundamentals of science in educating for social work practice. *Journal of Education for Social Work,* 2:22-29, 1966.

Ferster, C. B., and Skinner, B. F.: *Schedules of Reinforcement.* New York, Appleton-Century-Crofts, 1957.

Gelfand, D., and Hartmann, D.: Behavior therapy with children: A review and evaluation of research methodology. *Psychological Bulletin,* 69:204-215, 1968.

Gordon, W. E.: Basic constructs for an integrative and generative conception of social work. In G. Hearn (Ed.): *The General Systems Approach: Contributions Toward an Holistic Conception of Social Work.* New York, Council on Social Work Education, 1969.

Holland, J., and Skinner, B. F.: *The Analysis of Behavior.* New York, McGraw-Hill, 1961.

Hunt, J. McV.: Intrinsic motivation and its role in psychological development. In D. Levine (Ed.), *Symposium on Motivation.* Lincoln, University of Nebraska, 1965.

Maier, H. W.: *Three Theories of Child Development.* New York, Harper & Row, 1965.

McInnis, E. T.: Effects of Time-out and Response Cost Punishment Procedures upon Response Rate in Children, Unpublished doctoral dissertation. University of Illinois, 1969.

McQueen, M. M. *A Conceptual Framework for Testing the Patterns of Behavior Employed by Parents for Engaging in the Changing Process of the Child,* Doctoral dissertation, Washington University, Ann Arbor, Michigan, University Microfilms, 1965, No. 66-482.

McQueen, M. M. The role of the social worker in the remediation of children with learning disabilities. In *Patterns of Innovative Practice: School*

Social Work Conference. Springfield, Illinois, Department of Education, 1967, pp. 59-60.

Patterson, G. R., and Guillion, M. E.: *Living with Children: New Methods for Parents and Teachers.* Champaign, Illinois, Research Press, 1968.

Patterson, G. R., Jones, R., Whittier, J., and Wright, M.: A behavior modification technique for the hyperactive child. *Behaviour Research and Therapy,* 2:217-226, 1965.

Peterson, D. R.: *The Clinical Study of Social Behavior.* New York, Appleton-Century-Crofts, 1968.

Quay, H. C., Werry, J. S., McQueen, M. M., and Sprague, R. L.: Remediation of the conduct problem child in the special class setting. *Exceptional Children,* 32:509-515, 1966.

Redl, F., and Wineman, D.: *The Aggressive Child.* Glencoe, Illinois, Free Press, 1957.

Reidy, J.: *Zone Mental Health Centers: The Illinois Concept.* Springfield, Thomas, 1964.

Ullmann, L. P., and Krasner, L.: *A Psychological Approach to Abnormal Behavior.* Englewood Cliffs, N. J., Prentice Hall, 1968.

Werry, J. S., and Quay, H. C.: Observing the classroom behavior of elementary school children. *Exceptional Children,* 6:461-470, 1969.

Werry, J. S., and Wollersheim, J.: Behavior therapy with children: A broad overview. *Journal of the American Academy of Child Psychiatry,* 6:346-370, 1967.

APPENDICES

Appendix A

DESCRIPTION OF STAFF ROLES

APPENDIX A lists the duties and responsibilities for the Project Coordinator, Cottage Director, Extramural Case Coordinators, and the Intramural Counselors. There were, of course, many other people involved in the research project, and their functions are explained briefly in the text, where necessary. The author felt, however, that the functions divided between the positions described in this appendix were essential to the project.

PROJECT COORDINATOR

The Project Coordinator was a full-time professional employee who was paid from research funds. The functions of this position were as follows:

1. To act as Project Director in the absence of the Director.
2. To make substantial contributions to the program context and program evaluation.
3. To maintain a continuing staff-training program.
4. To supervise the development of each child's program.
5. To supervise the collection of data.

COTTAGE DIRECTOR

The Cottage Director was under the administrative direction of both the Adler Zone Center and the Children's Research Center. All clinical and programmatic research matters were reported by the Cottage Director directly to the Project Director, and all nonclinical and nonresearch matters were reported to Adler's Intramural Unit Manager. The functions of this position were as follows:

1. To supervise, under direction of the Project Director, the implementation of the research program as it applied to the total treatment program for the children, the collection of research data, and the activities of the child-care workers.
2. To meet regularly with the Project Director, to keep the Director informed on all problem areas and Adler policy and procedures, and to provide other feedback to the Director in order to insure smooth and effective functioning of the research program.
3. To meet regularly with the Intramural Unit Manager, to keep the Unit Manager informed on all problem areas, to consult with the Unit Manager on all matters of Adler policy and extraordinary procedures, and to review same periodically with the Unit Manager.
4. To work closely with other Adler personnel in evaluating therapeutic programs at all levels as required in order to insure the effective implementation of the research project.

5. To coordinate, plan, and supervise the implementation of all the activities for the cottage.

6. To assume responsibility for the care and appearance of the physical plant and equipment assigned to the program.

7. To conduct regular staff meetings to discuss program changes and problem areas, to inform staff of procedural revisions and their implementation, to make up work schedules and monitor work hours, and to review reports and other important areas of subordinates' work.

EXTRAMURAL CASE COORDINATORS

The Extramural Case Coordinators were professional staff members who were employed in the extramural division of the Adler Zone Center. Extramural Case Coordinators could be a psychiatrist, psychologist, social worker, special educator, or nurse. The functions of this position were as follows:

1. To introduce the case at the preadmission meeting for placement in Adler, including the preparation of case material for presentation.

2. To participate actively in the child's course of intramural care,
   a. facilitating a continuing relationship between the child and the community,
   b. developing a continuing treatment plan for the child in cooperation with the Project Director and/or Project Coordinator, Intramural Counselor, and appropriate school personnel.

3. To implement plans for the child's return to his home community or for his transfer to another type of service.

4. To contribute to the unit program development and evaluation.

INTRAMURAL COUNSELORS

The Intramural Counselors were Mental Health Workers, a state civil-service classification, who were employed by Adler and assigned to the project cottage. The functions of this position, before admission and during Orientation Level, were as follows:

1. To attend the admission conference on the child and to make a preadmission visit, if appropriate.

2. To post the Notice of Admission and the room assignment.

3. To orient the child to the unit—explain routine, rules, introduce the child to the kids and staff.

4. To make sure the clothing was marked.

5. To establish a relationship with the child.

6. To monitor the baseline data gathered during Orientation Level.

7. To arrange for any special observations.

8. To inform the staff of any special management orders effective immediately.

9. To check with the school regarding the testing schedule and to attend the school planning meeting.

10. To hold a pre-planning meeting during the first or second week of the child's residence in order to prepare for the treatment planning meeting.

11. To hold a treatment planning meeting and plan the child's program.

12. To write up the program for the cardex.

13. To notify the school when the program begins, to inform the teachers of the program, and to notify the teachers of any change in the program.

14. To complete the child's entrance records.

15. To monitor school during baseline in order to see that baseline recording of deviant behavior occurred.

16. To write up any special night procedures.

The Intramural Counselor's ongoing responsibilities were as follows:

1. To meet with the Assistant Counselor.

2. To record any special appointments, etc., on the calendar.

3. To post and date the staff slips, to monitor to see that all staff had read the material, and to remind them if necessary.

4. To prepare a prototype Mark Sheet and put it in the cardex and the night book, and to change both samples whenever there was a program change.

5. To keep the cardex, information sheet, night book, and the

school exchange sheet up to date, and also to inform the person in charge of these.

6. To monitor the data book.

7. To plan for home visits.

8. To determine the child's clothing and other basic needs and, if inadequate, to arrange with the Extramural Case Coordinator to obtain; if this was not possible, go through other Adler procedures to obtain.

9. To write the clinical-review report and to attend the Clinical Review Committee meeting.

10. To arrange for any special backups (trips, etc.) that were used in the child's program.

11. To arrange for coverage on the cottage at times when he was off for a period of time.

12. To contact the proper person to arrange for the child to go to public school; to meet with the public-school teachers or to establish some sort of regular communication system.

13. To work with the Extramural Case Coordinator on a home program—Intramural Counselor's responsibility and involvement in the home program varied.

14. To keep any data records relevant to the child's program.

15. To plan appropriate activities for the child's movement from one level to another.

16. To aid the Extramural Case Coordinator in working with family, public school, etc., and to make off-unit visits if necessary.

17. To meet with the Extramural Case Coordinator and teachers.

The Intramural Counselor's responsibilities that were related to discharge of the child were (a) to arrange for signing of the discharge forms and (b) to plan with the Extramural Case Coordinator and the Cottage Director for discharge.

Appendix B

INSTRUMENT SAMPLES

APPENDIX B provides samples of the instruments that are described in Chapter 4. They are arranged in the following order within the appendix:
Daily Checklist
Mark Sheets
    1. Time Out
    2. Response Cost
    3. School
Special Behavior Report Forms
    1. Time out with instructions for completion
    2. Response cost with instructions for completion
    3. Baseline (instructions for completion in Appendix C, Procedures for Orientation Level)
Independent Observations Handbook, plus examples of how behaviors fit into categories
Observer's Rating Sheet
Observer's Summary Sheet

DAILY CHECKLIST

ID (1-4)   DATE _____ (5-6)   MON ___ (7-8)   DAY ___ (9-10)   YEAR ___ (11-12)

CODE: 0 = Behavior not performed   X = No opportunity
        1 = Behavior performed   N = Not observed

Behavior												Col
Out of bed on time												13
Makes bed												14
Room neat												15
Closets and drawers neat												16
Dressed neatly												17
Hair neat												18
On time – breakfast												19
Appropriate table manners (B)												20
Appropriate social behavior (B)												21
Brush teeth (B)												22
Arrives in school on time												23
Wash hands before lunch												24
On time – lunch												25
Appropriate table manners (L)												26
Appropriate social behavior (L)												27
Brush teeth (L)												28
Arrives in school on time												29
Wash hands before dinner												30
On time – dinner												31
Appropriate table manners (D)												32
Appropriate social behavior (D)												33
Brush teeth (D)												34
Takes shower												35
Dressed appropriately for bed												36
Puts out laundry												37
In room at bedtime												38
Home, sick												39
ID												

Appendix B

MARK SHEET

Time-Out Punishment

ID_____ NAME_____ DATE_____

Total ASB Possible: Targets 1_____, 2_____, 3_____

_____Total School Possible   Total MAB Possible_____

ASB—1_____

			5			10
			15			20
			25			30
			35			40

SCHOOL

			5			10
			15			20
			25			30
			35			40

ASB—2_____

			5			10
			15			20
			25			30
			35			40

MAB

			5			10
			15			20
			25			30
			35			40

ASB—3_____

			5			10
			15			20
			25			30
			35			40

SAVINGS

ONE

			5			10
			15			20

FIVE

			5			10
			15			20

TEN

			5			10
			15			20
			25			30

ASB—4_____

			5			10
			15			20

STORE_____ OFF UNIT_____ HOME_____

PAID ON FINE_____

McQueen   8/8/69

[white]

MARK SHEET

Response-Cost Punishment

ID _____ NAME _____ DATE _____

Total ASB Possible: Targets 1_____, 2_____, 3_____

_____ Total School Possible   Total MAB Possible _____

ASB–1 _____

			5			10
			15			20
			25			30
			35			40

SCHOOL

			5			10
			15			20
			25			30
			35			40

ASB–2 _____

			5			10
			15			20
			25			30
			35			40

MAB

			5			10
			15			20
			25			30
			35			40

ASB–3 _____

			5			10
			15			20
			25			30
			35			40

SAVINGS

ONE

			5			10
			15			20

FIVE

			5			10
			15			20

ASB–4 _____

			5			10
			15			20

TEN

			5			10
			15			20
			25			30

STORE _____ OFF UNIT _____ HOME _____

PAID ON FINE _____   McQueen   8/8/69

[yellow]

Appendix B

MARK SHEET

School

ID _____ NAME _____ DATE _____

Rate of exchange for unit marks:

earned/poss.　　　unit marks poss.　　　unit marks given　　　special "things" poss. — earned?

		5			10
		15			20
		25			30
		35			40

		5			10
		15			20
		25			30
		35			40

		5			10
		15			20
		25			30
		35			40

		5			10
		15			20
		25			30
		35			40

		5			10
		15			20
		25			30
		35			40

NOTES:

		5			10
		15			20

TIME OUT: _____ MINUTES

Spaces are to be filled out by teacher.

[blue]

INSTRUCTIONS FOR FILLING OUT SPECIAL BEHAVIOR REPORT FORMS

Time Out

General Instructions

1. A form should be filled out each time a child spends time in TO.

It is possible that some children's programs may specify that TOs may be served in their rooms. Even if this is the case, a TO form should still be filled out each time the child is sent to his room.

If a child has been in TO, and misbehaves as he is coming out so that he is immediately returned to TO, it should be treated as a new incident and a new TO form filled out.

2. All of the information which is to be entered into boxes (ID ☐☐☐☐) is keypunched on IBM cards. It is important that numbers entered in the boxes be legible. If an error is made and you want to correct it, the number must either be erased or the incorrect number and its box scratched out and the correct number enclosed in a hand-drawn box on the same line as the original box (ID ~~0|0|1|1~~ |0|0|1|0|).

Information which is not entered in boxes is there for the benefit of the child-care staff and is not recorded as a formal part of the research data. While information such as the Behavior Description is not processed as data, this information is extremely useful to the Counselor and Coordinator and should routinely be filled out.

3. When entering data into the boxes, the number being entered should be placed as far to the right as possible and any unnecessary boxes should be filled with zeros (10 would be entered thus: |0|0|1|0|; 5 as |0|0|0|5|; 100 as |0|1|0|0|).

Specific Instructions

1. Identifying Information Required:
   a. Child's initials and ID Number (Only the ID Number is

Appendix B

absolutely required, but the initials are extremely helpful and should routinely be entered).

b. Month, day, year, time
March 23, 1970, 7:30 P.M. would be as follows:
Month $\boxed{0|3}$ Day $\boxed{2|3}$ Year $\boxed{7|0}$ Time $\boxed{2}$ $\boxed{0|7}$: $\boxed{3|0}$
A.M. = 1; P.M. = 2

c. Worker's ID Number. Use your Department of Mental Health number.

d. Location of offense
Forms now read: Unit staff = 1
School staff = 2
They will soon be changed to: Unit = 1
School = 2

If the offense occurred in the class room, it is considered a school contingency. If the offense occurred in the school hall or gym, a unit contingency is invoked and it is recorded as unit. There may be borderline cases where the offense occurs just as the child enters the classroom. In most cases, this would probably be considered a school offense, but workers will have to make a judgment depending upon the situation.

2. Initial Contingency:

Indicate which behavior first resulted in the application of a contingency. This should be a single behavior. A frequent error is to record the most serious deviant behavior in a chain of behaviors rather than the initial offense.

3. Misbehaviors Occurring after the Initial Behavior but before Entering the TO Room:

A series of boxes is provided where those behaviors which occur after the initial behavior may be recorded. There is also a place to record the number of times a specific deviant behavior occurred, or if it was a continuous behavior, the number of 15-second intervals during which it occurred. For example: If a child bit you four times on the way to the TO room, it would be recorded as

Behavior
Code Number
$\boxed{6|0|4}$

No. Occurrences
(15-second intervals)
$\boxed{0|4}$

If the child was verbally abusive during the time he was going to the TO room (say 3 minutes worth), it would be recorded as

Behavior Code Number	No. Occurrences (15-second intervals)
	3	0	3			1	2	

If the child hit you twice, then was verbally abusive for two minutes and then destroyed a game, it would be

Behavior Code Number	No. Occurrences (15-second intervals)
	6	0	4			0	2	
	3	0	3			0	8	
	5	0	6			0	1	

If a continuous act of deviant behavior occurs for more than 99 15-second intervals, for example, if defiance lasted for 120 15-second intervals (30 minutes), it would be recorded as

Behavior Code Number	No. Occurrences (15-second intervals)
	3	0	1			9	9	
	3	0	1			2	1	

4. Increasing Time in TO:

The amount of time a child must spend in TO is determined by the *highest level* deviant behavior he exhibits between the time a contingency is invoked and he enters the TO room. Thus, if the initial contingency was for a 101 but he commited a 303 on the way to TO, he would have to serve 30 minutes instead of 10 minutes.

If there is any misbehavior for which a contingency would ordinarily be invoked after the initial incident but before the child enters TO, then the time the child must stay in time out is increased by half.

Some examples:

If a 101 was the initial event and another 101 occurred on the way to TO, the child would serve 10 plus 5 or 15 minutes (his original time increased by half).

Appendix B 153

If a 101 was the initial event but a 301 occurred on the way, the child would serve 30 minutes.

If a 101 was the initial event but a 301 occurred on the way and this was followed by a 303, then the child would serve 30 plus 15 or 45 minutes (his original time would be determined by the 301, and it would be increased by half since deviant behavior continued to occur after the contingency for the 301 was invoked).

If a 301 was the initial event and two minutes of 304 occurred on the way to TO, the child would serve 30 plus 15 or 45 minutes. (30 minutes since it is the highest level increased by half since deviant behavior continued to occur. The frequency of the deviant behaviors on the way to TO does not result in any increase other than to increase the time by half.)

5. Delay before Entering the TO Room:

This is an indication of the time elapsed between the time you tell the child he must go to TO and the time the child enters the room.

6. Time Recycled, and Number of Times Recycled:

The time a child must serve does not start to count until he has quieted down (i.e. not yelling, kicking, etc.). If the child's time has begun but he then begins to cry and scream, his time is recycled, i.e. is begun again as soon as he quiets down.

Indicate whether the time was recycled or not, and if it was recycled, the number of times it was.

7. Time Spent in TO:

Indicate the total time spent in TO in minutes. An hour and 10 minutes would be $\boxed{0|0|7|0}$.

8. Time Child Gets Out of TO:

Indicate the time the child leaves the TO room. For example, 3:45 would be $\boxed{0|3}$: $\boxed{4|5}$.

SPECIAL BEHAVIOR REPORT FORM

TO   <u>TIME OUT</u>   **TO**

Child's Initials _____ ID ☐☐☐☐	Card Code ☐5☐1☐	1–6
Month ☐☐ Day ☐☐ Year ☐☐ Time ☐☐ : ☐☐		7–17
A.M. = 1		
P.M. = 2		
Worker ID ☐☐☐		18–20
Time Out ☐		21
Unit = 1 ☐		
School = 2		22

Behavior for which contingency is *initially* invoked ☐☐☐   23–25
Other behavior occurring before entering T.O. room:

Behavior Code Number	No. Occurrences (15 sec. intervals)	
☐☐☐☐☐☐☐☐☐☐	☐☐☐☐☐	26–30
		31–35
		36–40
		41–45
		46–50
		51–55
		56–60
		61–65

Time increased by half   YES = 1   ☐   66
                              NO   = 0

Delay before entering T.O. Room   ☐   67
    1 = 0–5 min   2 = 6–10 min   3 = 11–15 min   4 = 16–20 min   5 = 20+ min
Time enters room _____   T.O. Recycled YES = 1   ☐   68
Last Time recycled _____   NO   = 0
                        Number Times Recycled ☐☐   69–70
                 Time spent in T.O. (minutes) ☐☐☐☐   71–74

TIME Child gets out of T.O. room (finally)   ☐☐ : ☐☐   75–78

BEHAVIOR DESCRIPTION

Antecedent Events: _____

_____

Description of Behavior: _____

_____

Consequent Events: _____

                                                             McQueen   7/16/69

Appendix B 155

INSTRUCTIONS FOR FILLING OUT SPECIAL BEHAVIOR REPORT FORMS
Response Cost

General Instructions

1. A form should be filled out for each situation when a child is fined.

2. All of the information which is to be entered into boxes (ID |‾|‾|‾|‾|) is keypunched on IBM cards. It is important that numbers entered in the boxes be legible. If an error is made and you want to correct it, the number must either be erased or the incorrect number and its box scratched out and the correct number enclosed in a hand-drawn box on the same line as the original box (ID ~~|0|0|1|1|~~ |0|0|1|0|).

Information which is not entered in boxes is there for the benefit of the child-care staff and is not recorded as a formal part of the research data. While information such as the Behavior Description is not processed as data, this information is extremely useful to the Counselor and Coordinator and should routinely be filled out.

3. When entering data into the boxes, the number being entered should be placed as far to the right as possible and any unnecessary boxes should be filled with zeros (10 would be entered thus: |0|0|1|0|; 5 as |0|0|0|5|; 100 as |0|1|0|0|).

Specific Instructions

1. Identifying Information Required:
   a. Child's initials and ID Number (Only the ID Number is absolutely required, but the initials are extremely helpful and should routinely be entered).
   b. Month, day, year, time
      March 23, 1970, 7:30 P.M. would be as follows:
      Month |0|3| Day |2|3| Year |7|0| Time |2| |0|7| : |3|0|
           A.M. = 1
           P.M. = 2

c. Worker's ID number. Use your Department of Mental Health number.
d. Location of offense
   Forms now read: Unit staff = 1
                     School staff = 2
   They will soon be changed to: Unit   = 1
                                   School = 2

If the offense occurred in the classroom, it is considered a school contingency. If the offense occurred in the school hall or gym, a unit contingency is invoked and it is recorded as a unit. There may be borderline cases where the offense occurs just as the child enters the classroom. In most cases, this would probably be considered a school offense, but workers will have to make a judgment depending upon the situation.

2. Initial Contingency:

Indicate which behavior first resulted in the application of a contingency. This should be a single behavior. A frequent error is to record the most serious deviant behavior in a chain of behaviors rather than the initial offense.

3. Misbehaviors Occurring after the Initial Behavior:

A series of boxes is provided where those behaviors which occur after the initial behavior may be recorded. There is also a place to record the number of times a specific deviant behavior occurred, or if it was a continuous behavior, the number of 15-second intervals during which it occurred. For example: If a child bit you four times, it would be recorded as

Behavior	No. Occurrences
Code Number	(15-second intervals)
	6	0	4			0	4	

If the child was verbally abusive after a contingency is invoked (say 3 minutes worth), it would be recorded as

Behavior	No. Occurrences
Code Number	(15-second intervals)
	3	0	3			1	2	

Appendix B

If the child hit you twice, then was verbally abusive for two minutes and then destroyed a game, it would be

Behavior Code Number	No. Occurrences (15-second intervals)
	6	0	4			0	2	
	3	0	3			0	8	
	5	0	6			0	1	

If a continuous act of deviant behavior occurs for more than 99 15-second intervals, say for example defiance lasted for 120 15-second intervals (30 minutes), it would be recorded as

	3	0	1			9	9	
	3	0	1			2	1	

4. Lines are provided where staff may record the amount of the fine for each behavior. This is to make it easier to add up the total fine. It is not mandatory that these lines be used. Recording the total fine is necessary, however, and should be indicated in the boxes labeled "Total number of tokens fined."

5. In some cases of the punishable behavior may escalate until it is necessary to put the child in TO. If this occurs, then staff should indicate that TO was used as a backup, and the length of time the child spent in TO.

SPECIAL BEHAVIOR REPORT FORM

RC   RESPONSE COST   **RC**

Child's Initials _____ ID ☐☐☐☐	Card Code [5][1]	1–6
Month ☐☐ Day ☐☐ Year ☐☐ Time ☐☐:☐☐		7–17
	A.M. = 1	
	P.M. = 2	
Worker I.D. ☐☐☐		18–20
	Response Cost [0]	21
Unit = 1		
School = 2 ☐		22

Behavior for which contingency is *initially* invoked ☐☐☐   23–25
Other Deviant Behavior

Behavior Code Number	No. Occurrences (15 sec. intervals)	Amount of Fine	
☐☐	☐☐	_____	26–30
☐☐	☐☐	_____	31–35
☐☐	☐☐	_____	36–40
☐☐	☐☐	_____	41–45
☐☐	☐☐	_____	46–50
☐☐	☐☐	_____	51–55
☐☐	☐☐	_____	56–60
☐☐	☐☐	_____	61–65

Total number tokens fined   ☐☐☐☐   66–69

Back up T.O. used: YES = 1 NO = 0   ☐   70

Time spent in T.O. (minutes) ☐☐☐☐   71–74

BEHAVIOR DESCRIPTION

Antecedent Events: _____
_____
_____

Description of Behavior: _____
_____
_____

Consequent Events: _____
_____
_____

RC

McQueen   7/16/69

Appendix B

SPECIAL BEHAVIOR REPORT FORM
BASELINE

Child's Initials _____   ID [ ][ ][ ]   Card Code [6][1]   1– 6

Month [ ][ ]   Day [ ][ ]   Year [ ][ ]   7–12

Unit = 1
School = 2 [ ]   13

A	B	C	D	E	
					14–16
					17–19
					20–22
					23–25
					26–28
					29–31
					32–34
					35–37
					38–40
					41–43
					44–46
					47–49
					50–52
					53–55
					56–58
					59–61
					62–64
					65–67
					68–70
					71–73
					74–76

McQueen   2/24/69

INDEPENDENT OBSERVATIONS HANDBOOK
April, 1969

1. Definitions of Categories:
    a. Response Topography Dimension:
       This refers to what kind of response was made; i.e. what parts of the body were involved.
    b. Interaction Dimension:
       This refers to what people or objects were involved in the behaviors performed by the child being observed, i.e. what people or objects were acted on by child, or to what people the behavior was directed.
2. The Procedure will tell you how to record the symbols which are appropriate to what you have seen and heard.

RESPONSE TOPOGRAPHY CATEGORIES
Gross Motor Behaviors (G)

1. Movement of the whole body through space, e.g. walking, running, jumping, skipping, crawling, sliding, rolling, pulling self along, dancing, etc.

2. Activities which involve these movements a large part of the time but not all of the time will be rated under Gross Motor, e.g. playing Ping Pong, pool, flying a kit.

Kinds of Gross Motor Deviant Behavior

1. *Assaultive:* Movement of the entire body through space in the performance of hitting, kicking, biting, scratching, wrestling, pushing, pulling behaviors directed at other children and adults. Throwing objects would also be included if the child were also moving while throwing. There are many other kinds of assaultive behaviors which will be listed in the file. In general, however, for the behavior to be rated as Gross Motor Assaultive it must meet the basic definition of gross motor behavior—movement through space—and the definition of assaultive behavior—bringing some part of the body or another object into physical contact with another force.

2. *Defiance:* Any gross motor behavior which the child has just been requested or commanded not to engage in or whose proscription is a standing rule to be rated as gross motor defiance. Walking away from a staff member while he is speaking to the child is also gross motor defiance.

3. *Destructive:* Any gross motor behavior which is resulting in the damage to property is rated as destructive.

4. *Self-Destructive:* Any gross motor behavior resulting in damage or injury to the child engaging in the behavior is rated as self-destructive.

5. *Tantrum:* Any high intensity gross motor behaviors, such as kicking, stomping, pounding, jumping up and down, which are not being carried out as part of a game or sanctioned recreational activity.

Verbalizations (V)

1. Verbalizations include all audible vocal productions, e.g. speech, nonsense or other approximations to speech, grunts, groans,

and other vocal noises, screaming, crying, laughing.

2. It also includes visible movement of lips in the production of speech even though the sounds are not audible to the observer, e.g. children whispering to each other.

Kinds of Deviant Verbalizations

1. *Tantrum:* Screaming, yelling, and any other loud vocal production which are a part of a rage reaction.

2. *Defiance:* Verbal refusal to follow commands or to follow standing rule of conduct. Performance of verbal behaviors which have been countermanded, which would include obscenity, profanity, and proscribed topics.

3. *Antisocial:* Teasing and namecalling, bossing and criticizing behavior, verbal threats of physical harm, verbal blackmail or extortion, lying, bragging and boasting, tattling, and talking about others in a derogatory manner.

Fine Motor Behavior (F)

1. The distinction between Fine Motor and Gross Motor behaviors is that the child must be stationary in order for the behaviors to be classified as Fine Motor. The Fine Motor behaviors include observable movements made by distinct muscle groups, legs and feet, arms and hands, etc. and combinations of movements by these groups, while the person remains stationary, i.e. sitting, standing, prone, etc.

If the child is engaging in Gross Motor and Fine Motor behaviors consecutively, both can be rated.

If finer movements are being made while the child is also moving through space, the behavior is rated as a whole under Gross Motor, e.g. if child X is making an obscene gesture while jumping up and down, all the behaviors would be rated under Gross Motor Deviant.

Kinds of Fine Motor Deviant Behavior

1. *Assaultive*
2. *Destructive*
3. *Defiant*

For these three categories see the criteria listed under Gross Motor Deviant behaviors. Any behavior which satisfies the criterion for being fine motor and assaultive, destructive, or deviant would be rated as Fine Motor Deviant.

4. *Antisocial:* Any behavior which is fine motor and results in

cheating, teasing (use of gestures, funny faces, monster poses, imitations, etc.), and/or ignoring (turning away from someone speaking to child).

5. *Tantrums:* See Gross Motor Tantrum. This would also include sudden disruption of onging activity, i.e. child throws checkerboard to floor in the middle of the game.

Inactive (I)

1. If the child is not performing any gross motor, fine motor, or verbal behaviors, he is rated as Inactive. Movements of the eyes are not counted as fine motor behaviors.

Kinds of Deviant Inactive Behavior

1. *Ignoring:* The child makes no response at all to neutral or positive verbalizations addressed to him.

2. *Isolation:* The child is inactive and at least three feet away from the closest person.

3. *Teasing:* In certain cases a child may be teasing someone else only by the movement of his eyes. This would be rated as Inactive minus.

RESPONSE TOPOGRAPHY CATEGORIES

Staff Behaviors (S)

These are rated only when staff interacts with the child being observed so the interaction dimension need not be rated.

I. Approving Reactions (+)

Praise: Verbal approval or praise. Examples: That's good; You are doing well; I like the way you're working; you make me happy; Thank you; I like you; I like that.

Contact: Physical contact such as embracing, kissing, patting, holding arm or hand, having to sit in lap.

Approving head reactions: Smiling, winking, nodding. (Rate only if Praise is not rated.)

Granting privileges: Helping teacher; Choice of games; Doing something "first"; Choice of activity. (All response contingent.)

Promise of privilege: If occurs, note in comments.

II. Disapproving Reaction (—)

Critical verbal comment: Yelling, scolding, raising voice, screaming. Need not be of high intensity, e.g. Don't do that; Stop talking; Did I call on you; You are wasting your time; Don't laugh; Go to the office; You know what you are supposed to do.

Holding the child: Forcibly restraining child; forcibly removing child from room; grabbing, hitting, spanking, slapping, or shaking child.

Critical use of rules: You know we don't talk during work time.

Disapproving head reactions: Frowning, grimacing, side-to-side head shaking. (Not rated if "Critical verbal comment").

Threat of withholding privilege or of punishment: If—then statements of loss of privilege or punishment at some time in future.

Withholding privileges: Keeping in from recess (action); Depriving child of classroom privilege (specify).

Termination of social interaction: Turns out lights and says nothing; Turns back on class and waits for quiet; Stops talking and waits for quiet; Isolate from group.

Sending out of room: To hall, office, principal, etc. Note if occurs.

Stating rules: Any reminders of classroom rules asking a child to repeat the rule; Point to the rule on the board; etc. (Do not rate if "Critical use of rules" is rated.)

III. Neutral (0)

Do this: Giving instructions as to what to do. "Do this." "Turn to page x." Get out your books."

Explanation: Stating why things should be done a certain way; Giving reasons; Explaining meanings of concepts, etc.

Prompting: Help the child give the right answer with partial or total prompts.

Academic recognition: Call on child for an answer.

Probing: Asking questions to elicit information from child.

O.K. confirmation: That's right, O.K., marking correct, etc. (Do not rate if Praise is rateable).

Error: That's wrong, checking wrong, etc. (Do not rate if Critical verbal comment is rateable).

Other: Interacting with child, Can't tell if "Explanation" or "O.K. confirmation."

DEFINITIONS FOR INTERACTION DIMENSION

1. *Presence:* For the child to be in the presence of others, he must be within three feet of the closest person.
2. *Attention:* The child has the attention of someone else if any child or adult is watching what the child is doing.
3. *Directed at:* If the child has the attention of another person and is watching that person watch him, establishing eye contact with the person, or addressing the person, the child is directing behavior at the attending person. The child is directing behavior also if he calls the attention of another verbally or gesturally.
4. *Physical Contact:* This includes contact established by touching objects which both are holding, or by propelling objects between one another, as in Ping Pong or catch.

CRITERIA FOR THE INTERACTION DIMENSION

1. *Object:* Rate interaction with an object when the child is manipulating an object and is not directing his behavior at others or is not in physical contact with others.

Exception: When the child is participating in formal games like Monopoly and manipulating objects which are part of the game in the appropriate manner, rate interaction with whoever else is playing even though the others may not be paying attention. When the child is doing something by himself which involves the manipulation of objects, this interaction is rated as interaction with object.

2. *Self:* If the object of the behavior is a part of the child's body or if it involves just movements of his body and the behavior is not directed at anyone else and there is no physical contact with others, then the interaction is rated as self interaction.

3. *Peer:* If the behavior is addressed to or directed at or involves physical contact with another child, then it is rated as interaction with peer.

4. *Adult:* Same as for peer; substitute adult for peer.

5. *Adult and Peer:* If the behavior is directed at more than one person simultaneously and the group contains adults and peers, then it is rated interaction with adult and peers.

PROCEDURE

1. Watch child for nine seconds. Record behaviors one second. Rest the last 10 seconds of the minute.

2. After deciding what category the behavior falls under with respect to response topography (gross motor = G, fine motor = F, verbal = V, inactive = I) find the row which corresponds to that category. There will be one row of boxes on the rating sheet for each of the categories. Record the response by placing a number in the appropriate box. The number indicates what kind of interaction was involved (with peer and staff = 5; staff = 4, peer = 3, self = 2, object = 1).

3. If the behavior fell under one of the deviant subcategories, place a minus after the number. If the behavior is not deviant, it is considered appropriate and needs no further designation.

4. Use the special labels for the target behaviors. All target behaviors will be subsets of the four major respone-topography categories, and therefore should be placed in the row which corresponds to the more general category.

5. If both deviant and appropriate behaviors of the same topography occur in the same interval, record the deviant behavior, e.g. if child X has been carrying on a pleasant conversation for four seconds and then begins to swear, record the swearing, i.e. deviant verbal behavior for that interval.

Examples of how the concrete behaviors fitted into the observational categories:

Positive Staff Reaction
"You're being a good sport, Johnnie."
Negative Staff Reaction
"Johnnie, stop teasing Tommy."
Neutral Staff Reaction
"Johnnie, today is such a nice day."
Verbal (Objects)
    Deviant: Child is holding a ball. He says, "I am going to break the window with this ball."
    Nondeviant: Child is bouncing a ball. He counts, "One, two, three, four, five, six. . . ."
Verbal (Self)
    Deviant: Child is alone. He says, "I want to see a green car with a cracked window . . . etc."
    Nondeviant: Child in class. "One, two, three, take away two, one, two, is one."
Verbal (Peers)
    Deviant: Johnnie says, "Martha, you're a big fat pig."
    Nondeviant: Johnnie says, "Martha, may I play with you?"
Verbal (Staff)
    Deviant: Johnnie says, "I hope your baby dies."
    Nondeviant: Johnnie says, "Hi! I am glad to see you."
Verbal (Group)
    Nondeviant: Staff and children are at table working on arts and crafts.
    Johnnie says, "Somebody please pass the paste."
    Deviant: Same situation. Johnnie says, "Everyone here is a bastard."
Fine Motor (Objects)
    Deviant: Johnnie is sitting chipping away at the wall with a pencil.
    Nondeviant: Johnnie is sitting at his desk gluing a model together.

Fine Motor (Self)
  Deviant: Johnnie is sitting masturbating.
  Nondeviant: Johnnie is sitting down cutting his fingernails.
Fine Motor (Peers)
  Deviant: Johnnie is sitting next to Tommy and pinches him.
  Nondeviant: Johnnie is sitting playing checkers with Tommy.
Fine Motor (Staff)
  Deviant: Johnnie is making faces at staff.
  Nondeviant: Johnnie is sitting passing a piece of bread to staff.
Fine Motor (Group)
  Deviant: Johnnie is seated with adults and kids, playing a game and overturns the board knocking all pieces off.
  Nondeviant: Johnnie is seated with other children and staff playing Sorry.
Gross Motor (Objects)
  Deviant: Johnnie is jumping up and down on his bed.
  Nondeviant: Johnnie is jumping rope.
Gross Motor (Self)
  Deviant: Johnnie alone is jumping up and down, screaming, flailing air.
  Nondeviant: Johnnie is running laps in P.E.
Gross Motor (Peers)
  Deviant: Johnnie makes a flying tackle of Tommy as Tommy is walking across room.
  Nondeviant: Johnnie and Tommy are playing tag and Johnnie is chasing Tommy.
Gross Motor (Staff)
  Deviant: Johnnie runs up and pushes staff down.
  Nondeviant: Johnnie and staff are playing Duck, Duck, Goose.
Gross Motor (Group)
  Deviant: Johnnie grabs a ball the group is playing with and runs away.
  Nondeviant: Johnnie, staff, and other kids are playing musical chairs.
Inactive (Objects) Not observed
Inactive (Self)
  Deviant: Johnnie is sitting in room alone doing nothing during a structured activity period.
  Nondeviant: Johnnie is sitting still with eyes closed waiting for others to come outside.

Inactive (Peers)
  Deviant: Johnnie sits and ignores all verbal interactions directed to him by peers.
  Nondeviant: Johnnie sits waiting for his turn in a game with Tommy.
Inactive (Staff)
  Deviant: Johnnie sits and ignores staff verbalizations.
  Nondeviant: Johnnie stands still and lets staff part his hair.
Inactive (Group)
  Deviant: Johnnie is reading a comic while the group is waiting for him to make his move in a game.
  Nondeviant: Johnnie is in a game with adults and kids and is waiting his turn.

OBSERVER'S RATING SHEET

McQueen   3/7/69

Appendix B

OBSERVER'S SUMMARY SHEET

I.D. ☐☐☐	⟨5⟩⟨7⟩ Month ☐☐ Day ☐☐ Year ☐☐		1–12
Observer No. ☐	☐☐☐☐ Time	Unit = 1 School = 2 ☐	☐ 13–19
	☐☐☐☐ TOTAL		20–23
	☐☐☐ DEVIANT		24–26
	☐☐☐ RELIABILITY		27–29

	(+)	(−)	(0)		
S	☐☐☐	☐☐☐	☐☐☐		30–38

	(+)	(−)		(+)	(−)	
G	☐☐☐	☐☐☐	V	☐☐☐	☐☐☐	39–50
F	☐☐☐	☐☐☐	I	☐☐☐	☐☐☐	51–62
H2	☐☐☐	☐☐☐	3	☐☐☐	☐☐☐	63–74
4	☐☐☐	☐☐☐				75–80

Card 2

	(+)	(−)			⟨2⟩	19
5	☐☐☐	☐☐☐				20–25
	☐☐☐	☐☐☐	☐☐☐	☐☐☐		26–37
	☐☐☐	☐☐☐	☐☐☐	☐☐☐		38–49
	☐☐☐	☐☐☐	☐☐☐	☐☐☐		50–61
	☐☐☐	☐☐☐	☐☐☐	☐☐☐	−	62–73

McQueen 4/10/69

Appendix C

PROCEDURES AND POLICIES

APPENDIX C CONTAINS the procedures and policies used in the research project. They are arranged in the following order within the appendix:

1. Orientation Level.
2. Daily Schedule of Activities.
3. List of Backups.
4. Punishment Contingencies.
5. Time-out Procedures.
6. Response-Cost Procedures.

PROCEDURES AND POLICIES FOR THE ORIENTATION LEVEL

Data Recording

1. Child-care workers are to record all incidents of punishable behavior, as defined in punishment contingencies, on the Special Behavior Report Form-Baseline. This is done by simply listing the code number that indicates the punished behavior. A new Special Behavior Report Form-Baseline should be filled out for each day that a child spends on the Orientation Level. If no incidents of punishable behavior occur during that day, then "none" should be written on that sheet and a new one started for the next day. The baseline forms are to be left in the box for the Project Secretary at the end of the day.

If the child-care worker feels that the Intramural Counselor should have additional information regarding either the punished behavior or the situation in which it occurred, including the antecedent event, behavior, and consequences, then a behavior description should be prepared and put in the Counselor's box.

> NOTE: Teachers fill out a Special Behavior Report Form-Baseline for each child while he is on Orientation Level. These forms are to be picked up by a child-care worker from the school office at the end of the school day. The teachers have been asked to turn one in every day. If there were no incidents of punishable behavior, they should turn in a sheet marked "none." It may be necessary to remind teachers about filling out and turning in these sheets.

Child-care workers are to record potential reinforcers for the child on a sheet posted in the office (usually on the child's locker). This information would be obtained through observing talking with the child, or simply asking him about the kinds of things he likes.

3. Child-care workers are to record any behaviors that they feel might be a potential target. This is to be done on a sheet posted in the office (usually on the child's locker).

4. Any information that a child-care worker feels should be documented for the Counselor can be recorded on a Behavior Description Form and put in the Counselor's box.

5. Marks spent and the reinforcer purchasers are to be indicated on the child's Mark Sheet as they are spent.

6. Performance of the behaviors on the Daily Checklist is recorded in the regular manner.

Punishment Procedures

100-500 Level Behaviors

Staff is to *ignore* the occurrence of these behaviors. When the frequency and/or intensity of these behaviors is such that the staff member has reached the *limit* of his tolerance, then he may take whatever steps he feels are necessary, as long as TO is not used. Procedures that are to be used in these situations are deliberately not spelled out in order to avoid the systematic use of any one procedure. Each staff member is to do "his own thing" in these situations. Situations where the staff feel they can not continue to ignore the punishable behaviors should not be very frequent.

600 Level Behaviors

Use physical restraint (if necessary) and up to 50 minutes in TO. The child need not be left in TO for the full 50 minutes if he calms down sooner (the child-care worker is to use his judgment about the length of time). After 50 minutes, the child is to be let out of TO even if he has not calmed down. If the behavior is repeated, he is returned to TO for what may be another 50-minute TO. Major Destruction is also handled in this manner.

700 Level Behaviors

Counselors are to specify how these behaviors are to be dealt with in each individual case.

Lesser forms of assault and destruction may be handled by using physical intervention and restraint (if necessary), but TO should not be used in these cases. Staff may use whatever procedure (other than TO) they feel comfortable with in the situation. (See section on 100-500 Level Behaviors.)

Prices

Prices are arbitrarily set as five marks per item or event. Things that are rented for a period of time are generally five per one-half hour. The actual price is relatively unimportant; what we are really interested in finding out is how frequently the child chooses to take advantage of the things available to him. A list of some common prices follows, but if the child expresses interest in something for which no price had been set, just charge five marks.

Meals	5
T.V.	5 per ½ hour
Game Room	5 per ½ hour
Games	5 per ½ hour
Cart	5 per ½ hour
Phone Calls	5
Library Rental	5 per 24 hours
Off Unit	5 per ½ hour
Outside Play	5 per ½ hour
Unit Parties	5
Record Player	5 per ½ hour

During Orientation Level, the child is limited to 10 marks in the store per day. If the child wanted to purchase something that cost more than 10 marks, he can put marks toward it each day until it is paid for.

Off-unit

Off-unit activities are restricted to one during the week and one per weekend. Off units are any activity which takes place off the grounds of the Adler Zone Center.

Home Visits

Home visits are not available to those on orientation, except under unusual circumstances. Parents may visit during this time, if the arrangements are cleared with the child's Extramural Coordinator and Intramural Counselor.

Treats

There will be a limit of three treats (ice cream, oranges, apples, potato chips, etc.) per day while on orientation. Counselors may reduce this number if they feel that this is too many for their particular child.

Lost Mark Sheets

1. If a new sheet has to be issued, then the child can have 20 marks for the rest of the day. No additional marks could be given in this case.

2. If the original sheet is found after a new one has been issued, then the child receives a bonus of ten or more marks on the new sheet. All other marks on the original sheet are forfeited.

3. If a Mark Sheet is misplaced and recovered by staff (when it is carelessly left lying around and staff takes it to the office), all but 30 of the unspent marks are to be marked off as a recovery fee. A note should be made on the sheet indicating that no more marks are to be given for the rest of the day.

General Policies and Procedures

In general, with the exception of some deviant behaviors, no contingencies are applied either for the performance or nonperformance of any behavior. Prompts can be given in an effort to inform the child of our general expectations, i.e. "children here usually pick up their toys, make their beds, take a shower, come to meals on time," etc. There will be some "natural" contingencies that will follow some behaviors, i.e. not deciding to go skating until after the group has gone will mean missing the activity; coming to meals after kitchen staff has left the cottage will result in a missed meal. There will be, of course, more borderline situations where the staff will have to make a judgment. If a child is only a few minutes late to the meal, he may be served as usual, but if he is very late, he may miss part of it. Just how these borderline "natural" contingencies are to be handled will have to be decided by staff in the situation.

Some Specific Policies

1. Children who are ten years or older may stay up a half hour later (7 days a week) by paying five marks.

2. Younger children may not operate the record player while on Orientation Level.

3. When children are visiting in another's room, they may not close the door. Counselors can decide whether this policy will continue on Level I.

1/20/69 McQueen/McInnis

DAILY SCHEDULE OF ACTIVITIES

The following schedule is being instituted for several reasons, but the most basic is to provide more structure for both staff and children.

The basic notion is to restrict the number of activities which will be available during certain times of the day. The rationale for this is as follows:

1. Restriction of activities will alleviate some of the pressure on the staff to cover a "multitude" of activities simultaneously.
2. Staff assignments can be made ahead of time so that individual responsibilities can be well defined and there need be no anxiety about "who is doing what and what am I to do?"
3. Possible therapeutic effect upon the kids. It is expected that there will be more "wholesome" group experiences and less just "hanging around."
4. Enhancement of the reinforcing value of the activities. Since they will not be available at all times, there will be less satiation. Over time the kids may actually experience a wider range of activities, since they may choose a less desirable (from their point of view) activitiy in a situation where their favorite activity is not available.

There are two schedules proposed for evenings. One for the nights when there is an off-unit activity (possibly Monday, Wednesday, and one weekend night) and the other for evenings when there is a planned group activity (Tuesday, Friday, and one weekend night). Thursdays may necessitate a special schedule for those times when the party is not plugged in as a planned group activity, i.e. when the party occurs at supper or snack time. The activity therapist will be responsible for planning the off-unit and group activities. Staff who have ideas or suggestions about activities should feel free to tell them to this person.

DAY SHIFT

9:00 A.M.–3:00 P.M.   School and School breaks
School breaks may be either free time, lunch, or for some children may provide an opportunity for one-to-one sessions aimed at a particular problem, i.e. grooming, athletic skill, visits to Extramural Coordinators.

Before 3:00 P.M.   Children are to deposit their school Mark Sheet in the "Cottage G Mailbox." These will be removed at 3:15, and the staff will compute the number of spendable marks each child earned. A summary sheet will be available to record the number of marks each child is to be given. The marks will be given after PE. If the school sheet is not left in the box, the child will not be able to receive his school marks until some time after dinner, but before 6:30 P.M.

EVENING SHIFT

Off-unit Nights   **Group Activity Nights**

3:00–4:00   *Physical Education*
One staff from the evening shift covers at three o'clock. The others cover after report as needed. The number of staff needed to cover each PE activity will be indicated on the weekly activity schedule.

4:00–4:15   Give school marks and give out cold drinks certificates earned in PE.

Cold Drink Time

Those earning certificates get a free drink, others can buy one as a treat. The only treat available at this time is a cold drink.

4:15–5:00   *Activity Time**
Available: 1. TV   2. Outside or Activity Room
(whichever most people choose)

5:00–5:45   *Dinner*

5:45–6:20   *Activity Time**
Available during this time:
1. Outside (Bikes, skates, etc. can be used whenever outside is scheduled.)
2. Activity Room
3. Game Room (Record player will be kept in the game room unless staff decides to make it available in the activity room. It can be used in this way to reward the group when things have been going well.)

6:20   Those going off unit clean up and pay their marks.

6:30–7:15   *Quiet Time — Study Hall*
In the east dining room, books, magazines, art supplies, etc., will be available for those who do not have homework. All will be expected to work quietly on something. This may also be a time when some children may be scheduled for one-to-one sessions.

6:55   Those going off unit leave study hall.
7:00–8:30   *Off-Unit Activity**
7:15–7:30   Store and Treat Time
(for those not going off unit)

7:30–8:00   *Activity Time**   *Planned Group Activity*
1. Outside in defined play area. (Alternative is activity room if weather is bad or if short staffed.)

Appendix C 181

8:00–8:30 Little Kids — Shower
(When they finish their showers, they can stay in their room area until snack time.)
Big Kids Game Room (Those not playing watch or have quiet time in the east dining room.)   Continuation of planned activity with the Big Kids.

8:30–8:50 *Snacks*
9:00   Bedtime for Little Kids
Shower for Little Kids who went off unit.

8:50–9:30   Shower for Big Kids
9:30   Big Kids in bed or quiet in room
Bedtime for Little Kids who went off unit.

10:00   Bedtime for Big Kids

*NOTE: Whenever staff is short, one activity can be eliminated. There may also be times when off units cannot be offered even though scheduled because of staff shortages. In these cases, the staff may want to substitute a group activity and follow the group activity schedule.

Kids are to be encouraged to participate in the available activies even if they just watch. If a child refuses to do this, he is to stay in his room until the activity is over.

Phone calls can be scheduled any time the staff can handle them, except during study hall.

LIST OF BACKUPS

Arts and crafts supplies	Meals:	Party (Thursday)
	Breakfast	
Baking	Lunch	Phone calls
	Dinner	
Bedtime story		Record players

	Off units:	
Books	Bowling	Room visit
	Eat out	
Cold drink (after school)	Golf	Snacks
	Horse ride	
Comics	Movies	Special (Individual)
	Van ride	
Game room	Ice skating	Store
	Swimming	
Games	Bikes	T.V.
	Cart	
Gym	Just outside	Treats
	Skates	
Home visits	Walks	Up late
		Y.M.C.A.

PUNISHMENT CONTINGENCIES

100 Level

The time-out (TO) contingency to be used at this level is *10 minutes*. Response-cost fines are based on earning power. For earning power of less than 51 marks, the fine is 1 mark; for 51 to 85, 2 marks; for 86-115, 3 marks; and for earning above 115, 4 marks.

101—Defiance of Minor Rules and Requests

Defiance of rules at this level consists of the violation of those rules which are minor in the sense that their violation has relatively little consequence to the functioning of the cottage.

Examples of rules at this level:
1. Running ahead of staff (without permission) on the way to school.
2. Excessive noise in the school building (in the hall between classes).
3. Playing ball in the cottage.
4. Talking while at the Free Meal Table.

Defiance of requests has two relevant dimensions to be considered when invoking contingencies.
1. The first is in terms of the kind of behavior that the

Appendix C

child is requested to stop. At this level, the kinds of behavior which the child is requested to stop are those that are annoying, mildly disruptive, or that might possibly lead to more unacceptable behavior.
2. The second dimension to be considered is how the child responds to the request. If the child immediately complies with the request, no contingency is invoked. If the compliance is not immediate but only after the child engages in the behavior "one more time," then a Level 100 contingency would be invoked.

The behavior which a child is requested to stop may be appropriately placed at this level, but if the child's response is more directly defiant than described above, then a higher level contingency would be invoked. (See defiance at Level 200 and Level 300).

Examples of requests at this level:
1. A child is tattling on another child in a loud, harping fashion and is asked to quiet down.
2. A child is making noise or talking loudly and is asked to quiet down or stop. This request might be made of a child in the school building, if he was making too much noise, but it was not considered to be "excessive."
3. A child forgets to clear his own table service after a meal and is reminded that he should do so.
4. A child is "roughhousing" with another child and is asked to stop.
5. A child is asked to pick up or straighten up after an activity.

102—Minor-Moderate Tantrums

These are defined as inappropriate physical and verbal behavior of anger or frustration. They would include such behaviors as screaming, stamping feet, striking out, pounding on things, running around, throwing something on the floor, etc.

To be classed as a mild tantrum, the behavior exhibited

would have to be relatively mild in intensity and of relatively short duration.

> NOTE: Whining behavior by itself would not be considered a tantrum behavior. Whining might best be handled by ignoring, diverting, etc., or if these are not seen as appropriate, then by requesting that the whining cease.

103—Minor-Moderate Verbal Abuse

1. Inappropriate verbalizations directed toward adults.
    Examples: "Go to . . ."
    "Skip you."
    "Forget you."
    "Shut up."
    "Ugly!"
    "Sassing" might also be included

The same class of verbal behaviors would be considered to be Severe Verbal Abuse and result in a Level 300 contingency, if it was judged (from the context and emotional content) that the verbalization constituted a direct threat to adult authority.

2. Teasing, taunting, mocking, heckling, etc. (directed toward either a child or an adult).
    Derogatory name chanting
    Ridiculing—gestural or verbal

104—Minor-Moderate Physical Abuse

1. Physical pawing of staff or children (if told not to).
2. Physical teasing, i.e. poking, prodding, tickling, etc. (if requested to cease).

200 Level

The TO contingency at this level is *20 minutes*. For earning power of less than 51 marks, the fine is 2 marks; for 51-85, 4 marks; for 86-115, 6 marks; and for earning more than 115, 8 marks.

201—Defiance of More Serious Rules and Requests

Defiance of rules at this level consists of violation of rules which are more serious in the sense that their violation has greater consequence for cottage functioning than is the case at the 100 Level.

Examples of rules at this level:
1. Leaving the dining room before the end of the meal.
2. Using the Men's and Women's restroom in the school.
3. Climbing on the partitions in the washroom.
4. Climbing on the window ledges.
5. Coming out of their room in the morning before the designated time (except for going to the bathroom during the night).
6. Being in a restricted area. (Example: Being in the cupboards or closets in the activity room.)

Defiance of requests again has two relevant dimensions, the kind of behavior that the child is engaged in and how he responds to the request, which need to be considered in defining defiance at this level.

At this level, the kinds of behaviors the child is requested to stop are those which have greater consequence for cottage functioning or staff authority than is the case at the 100 Level.

In terms of the child's response to the request, defiance at this level would take the form of noncompliance or a simple refusal to comply with the request.

The kind of behavior that a child is requested to stop might be a 100 Level behavior, but if the child's response is noncompliance or a simple refusal to comply with the request, then a 200 Level contingency is invoked.

Examples of requests at this level:
1. A child does not respond to a request to leave a game because his behavior has been inappropriate.
2. A child does not return something to another child after being requested to do so. (This is distinct from stealing in that the child has openly come into possession of something that belongs to someone else.)

205—Lying

This was defined as the deliberate distortion of the truth to gain something for himself. This would not include exaggeration or "tall tales."

> NOTE: If a clear-cut behavior was observed and staff invokes a contingency, but the child denies that he performed this behavior, then the child is subject to a lying contingency. In this case, the child's denial would have to be considered as a definite lie and not a question of misperception on the part of the child. If this situation occurred in the RC condition, this would mean an additional fine; or in the TO condition, the time would be increased by half.

> NOTE: Cheating (in games and group activities) has not been included in the contingency system. Cheating is to be handled by asking the child to sit out for awhile. Staff will make a judgment concerning the length of time, etc., in terms of what seems to be appropriate in each individual case.

213—Attempted Provocation

This is defined as trying to elicit misbehavior from another but without success.

Examples of such behavior are:
1. A says to B, "C says bad things about you; why don't you hit her?"
2. One child urges another to break a rule—such as going into a restricted area.

> NOTE: If the provoker is successful, then he receives the same penalty as that received by the child provoked, unless the penalty is less than that for attempted provocation.

300 Level

The TO contingency at this level is *30 minutes*. For earning power of less than 51 marks, the fine is 4 marks; for 51-85, 8 marks; for 86-115, 12 marks; and for earning more than 115, 16 marks.

301—Defiance of Major Rules and Requests

Defiance of rules at this level consists of the violation of rules which are of major consequence in the sense that their violation is considered to be potentially more dangerous or disruptive.

Examples of rules at this level:
1. Leaving their room after bedtime (except for going to the bathroom).
2. Leaving the cottage without permission.
3. Violation of the room restriction. (See Procedure Book for current room restriction policy.)
4. Violation of the hall restriction (nonresidents entering the East Hall).
5. Locking the bathroom door of the Men's or Women's restroom in the school building.

Defiance of requests:

At this level, the kinds of behaviors that the child is requested to stop are those which are regarded as potentially dangerous to themselves or others, potentially destructive, and/or potentially disruptive to an ongoing activity.

Failure to comply with requests to cease this kind of behavior would result in invoking a contingency at this level.

Direct defiance of staff authority, a "you can't make me" response, would also result in a contingency at this level, even though the behavior involved would be appropriately placed at a lower level.

Examples of requests at this level:
1. A child is requested to stop using a toy in a dangerous manner (swinging a bat when others are near) or using potentially dangerous toys in an inappropriate manner (shooting arrows when others are in the vicinity).

302—Severe Tantrum Behavior

Inappropriate verbal and/or physical expression of anger or frustration is considered severe tantrum behavior.

At this level, the tantrum behavior would be of greater intensity, of longer duration, or would consist of a wider range of inappropriate behaviors.

> NOTE: A single behavior (such as screaming) of high intensity or long duration would be considered a severe tantrum.

303—Severe Verbal Abuse
   Objectionable ethnic names.
   Lewd and obscene comments. Example: "Go stick it up her ..."
   Obscene gestures, such as "the finger."
   Verbalizations which (judging from the context and emotional level) represent a direct threat to adult authority.

304—Minor Assault (On Children)
   Shoving, pushing, grabbing, holding.

305—Attempted Framing
   A child attempts to get a contingency invoked on another child by setting up a situation which makes it appear as though the other child had committed the deviant behavior.

> NOTE: If the deviant behavior in question has a more serious contingency, then the more serious contingency is invoked against the "framer."

> Example: If a child pours shampoo under another child's bed to make it appear as though that child had urinated in his room, then the framer would receive an 80 minute or 8 marks penalty instead of 40 minutes or 4 marks.

306—Minor Destruction of Property
   This is a case where the property destroyed is of relatively little value (pencil, piece of chalk, etc.), when the destruction results in little inconvenience or disruption to others, and where the emotional content of the action is relatively mild (on the part of the actor).

317—Threatening (Staff or Children)
   These are gestures or verbalizations which imply danger or harm to the individual (as opposed to gestures of a kidding or nonserious nature).
   Gestures would be considered threatening if they take place in close proximity to another person (example, punching motions made in someone's face).
   Throwing gestures, that are made with an object in hand, if

they are directed at an individual, would also be considered threatening.

400 Level

The TO contingency at this level is *40 minutes*. For earning power of less than 51 marks, the fine is 8 marks; for 51-85, 16 marks; for 86-115, 24 marks; and for earning more than 115, 32 marks.

407—Verbal Extortion and Bribery

1. Verbal extortion—coercing someone, extracting favors or material objects from someone by using threats (not necessarily threats of bodily harm).
>Example: "If you don't give me candy, I'll see to it that no one plays with you."

2. Bribery—giving something to someone or doing something for someone to get them to do some behavior which is not appropriate.
>Examples: A child giving someone else some candy so that they won't tell that he had violated the room restriction.
>A child giving someone a comic book to get them to back him up on some story (i.e., give him an alibi).

409—Urinating or Defecating in a Place Other Than the Designated Receptacles
>NOTE: Soiling behavior and bed wetting is not included in this category.

410—Child Leaves the TO Room Without Permission

411—A Child Talks to a Child Who Is in TO

412—Tearing Up a Door Chart

413—Aiding and Abetting Another's Misbehavior by Impeding Staff
>Examples: A child standing in the staff's way when he is going to deal with a stiuation

A child holding a door when a staff is trying to enter a room to intervene in trouble.

500 Level

The TO contingency at this level is *50 minutes*. For earning power of less than 51 marks, the fine is 12 marks; for 51-85, 24 marks; for 86-115, 36 marks; and for earning more than 115, 48 marks.

504—Assault

Physical attack upon another child (hitting, kicking, biting, etc.)

505—Forgery
    Examples: Altering Mark Sheet
                     Altering or making notes sent from or to school

506—Serious Destruction of Property

This involves the destruction of property of greater value (either monetary or personal value); the destruction results in disruption or inconvenience to others; or the emotional content of the act is relatively intense. This includes destruction of another child's Mark Sheet.

507—Extortion Through Use of Physical Force

520—Possession of Forbidden, Harmful, or Dangerous Items

521—Stealing

525—Inappropriate Sexual Behavior
    Examples: Public masturbation
                     Fondling another's genitals
                     Deliberate exhibitionism

Special Contingency Behaviors

Certain behaviors will be regarded as special in the sense that they will be handled outside of the system outlined above and will result in special contingencies that will be decided individually for each child. The Counselor will be responsible for seeing that the contingencies for 600 and 700 Level behaviors are specified in the child's program.

600 Level

604—Assault on an Adult
610—AWOL
699—Entering the Cottage Office

700 Level

706—Self-Destructive Behavior
709—Soiling Behavior
7—Idiosyncratic Deviant Behavior

TIME-OUT (TO) PROCEDURES

It is to be stressed that the staff members are to use all their skill to preclude the occurrence of behaviors which would require a punishment contingency. The punishment system is not seen as the only means of controlling inappropriate behavior. The punishment contingencies should be used only if other techniques (diversion, positive prompts, initiation of incompatible behaviors, etc.) have failed to prevent the occurrence of the inappropriate behavior.

If a behavior has occurred for which a contingency is necessary, then:

1. Inform the child of the contingency and the behavior for which it was invoked. This should be done in a matter-of-fact manner and with a neutral rather than a negative tone.

In the same manner (matter-of-fact neutral tone), the child should be given the prompt that if the behavior continues his time will be increased.

2. Take the child to TO. The location depends upon where the behavior occurred and the length of the TO period.

School

When ten- and twenty-minute penalties are involved in the school, the school TO room should be used. If the penalty is for more than twenty minutes, the child is returned to the cottage.

If both school TO rooms are in use, as an alternative, the child may be asked to sit in a chair facing the wall. When the child is serving a TO penalty in this fashion, if he calls out or talks to others in the hall, he should be returned to the cottage TO room where his time would begin again. This same procedure should be followed if the child continually turns around to look at the hall activity after a prompt has been given. Staff should be reasonable when considering returning a child for looking around and should take the circumstances into account, i.e., if there is a great deal of commotion in the hall, it would be unreasonable to expect that a child would not look to see what it was.

If the child behaves in any other inappropriate way while in the TO area, he would be sent back to the cottage. If these behaviors would result in a more severe contingency, then the penalty for those behaviors is invoked and this time is served in the cottage TO room.

If other Cottage G children talk to or tease, etc. a child in the TO area, then they should be sent to the cottage TO room for a ten-minute period.

Cottage

If both cottage TO rooms are in use, then it will be necessary to use the dining rooms and any empty bedrooms (in that order of priority). When using the empty bedrooms, make sure that the mattresses are standing on end and tell the child that he is not permitted to lie on them.

If a ten-minute penalty is invoked when the child is some distance from the cottage, a makeshift TO may be set up (taking the child away from the group and having him sit with his back to the group). When twenty-minute penalties are invoked some distance from the cottage, it will be up to the staff whether a child is returned to the cottage or not. But if penalties greater than twenty minutes are invoked, then the child should be returned, if possible, to the cottage TO room.

3. If the child does not respond appropriately when the con-

tingency is invoked (i.e., fails to stop the behavior and quiet down) or if he misbehaves while on the way to TO, then the length of time he is to spend in TO is increased by half (a ten-minute penalty would become fifteen minutes, etc.).

If a child acts upon the way to TO by emitting behaviors that are more serious than the one for which he is being punished, then the penalty for the more serious behavior is invoked.

4. If the child has not quieted down when he enters TO, the TO will not be started until he does so, or if he acts up after the time has been started, then his time will be recycled.

If the child emits behaviors in the TO room which have more serious consequences than the one for which he has been penalized, then the contingency for the more serious offense will be invoked.

5. A child may go to the bathroom once during a 30-, 40-, or 50-minute TO period (this is without being recycled). They can not leave to go to the bathroom during a 10- or 20-minute TO without being recycled.

6. A Special Behavior Report Form will be filled out each time a contingency is invoked indicating the behavior which led to the penalty, what penalty is invoked, and the child's reaction to the TO.

4/28/69 McQueen

RESPONSE-COST (RC) PROCEDURES

It is to be stressed that the staff members are to use all their skill to preclude the occurrence of behaviors which would require a punishment contingency. The punishment system is not seen as the only means of controlling inappropriate behavior. The punishment contingencies should be used only if other techniques (diversion, positive prompts, initiation of incompatible behaviors, etc.) have failed to prevent the occurrence of the inappropriate behavior. Response cost (RC) is to be used for those behaviors that are defined on the 100-500 Levels. RC may or may not be used for the 600 and 700 Level behaviors. This will be decided in each case by the Counselor.

If a behavior occurs for which a contingency is necessary then:

1. Inform the child of the contingency and the behavior for which it was invoked. This should be done in a matter-of-fact manner and with a neutral rather than a negative tone. In the same matter-of-fact manner, the child should be given the prompt that if the behavior continues it will be necessary to fine him again.

2. Mark the fine off on the Mark Sheet. If the child does not have his Mark Sheet with him or if he refuses to pay the fine, then tell the child that his fine will be noted on his balance sheet in the office and that he can pay it later.

> NOTE: Children will not be allowed to spend marks for anything else until they have paid their fine.

3. If the same class of behavior continues after the invoking of a fine, the child is fined again. This fine would be imposed if at least a fifteen-second interval had passed since the first fine. For behaviors which are continuous (strings of profanity, tantrums, etc.) rather than discrete, responses will be defined in terms of fifteen-second intervals. That is, each fifteen-second interval of such behavior will be counted as a single response and, therefore, subject to a fine. These fifteen-second intervals need not be timed with a watch, but the staff should practice judging fifteen-second intervals so that they can make fairly accurate judgments in the situation.

4. Each child on RC will have a fine base which is based on his potential earning power as defined in his program. The number of marks he is fined is computed by multiplying this base times the number assigned to each of the behavioral levels:

$100 = 1$ $300 = 3$ $500 = 5$
$200 = 2$ $400 = 4$

Thus, if a child had a fine base of 3 and he was being fined for a 300 Level behavior, he would pay 12 marks; for a 500 Level behavior, he would pay 36 marks, etc.

5. A special report form will be filled out each time that a contingency is invoked describing the behavior which led to the penalty, what penalty was invoked, and the child's reaction to the penalty. If a series of fines is invoked for the same class of

behavior, only one form need be filled out, but it should contain complete information regarding the behaviors and the fines invoked.

Recording of Fines and Their Payment

Each child will have a balance sheet in the office. This sheet will contain a column for fines, one for fine payments, and another for the running total.

All fines and payments will be recorded on this sheet, and the running total figured each time an entry is made.

Special Note

If a child is performing some behavior that cannot be allowed to continue (such as repeatedly hitting someone, destroying property, etc.), then physical intervention would be required. This would mean that the child would physically be prevented from continuing the activity. In some cases, it might be necessary to continue the physical restraint until the child has quieted down and regained control.

4/28/69 McQueen

Appendix D

SUPPLEMENTAL INFORMATION FOR ONE INDIVIDUAL PROGRAM

Appendix D contains supplemental information for one individual program presented in Chapter 7. Sample mark sheets and cardex material for all levels of Subject 19's program are arranged in the following order within the appendix:

Level I
Mark Sheet
Cardex
Level II
Mark Sheet
Cardex
Level II Phase II
Mark Sheet
Cardex
Level II Phase III
Mark Sheet
Cardex
Level III
Cardex
Home Visit Forms

MARK SHEET

ID _____19_____ NAME _____H.L.____ DATE **LEVEL I** _____

Total ASB Possible: Targets 1: _25_ , 2: _5_ , 3: _10_

_20_ Total School Possible   Total MAB Possible _____

ASB–1: **BEING NICE TO OTHER KIDS**   SCHOOL

		5			10
		15			20
		25			30
		35			40

		5			10
		15			20
		25			30
		35			40

ASB–2: **COOPERATION**   MAB

		5			10
		15			20
		25			30
		35			40

		5			10
		15			20
		25			30
		35			40

ASB–3: **GENERAL**   SAVINGS

		5			10
		15			20
		25			30
		35			40

ONE
		5			10
		15			20

FIVE
		5			10
		15			20

ASB–4:

		5			10
		15			20

TEN
		5			10
		15			20
		25			30

STORE_____   OFF UNIT_____   HOME_____
PAID ON FINE_____   McQueen   8/8/69

[yellow]

LEVEL I PROGRAM – HARRISON L.
(Program to begin 6/29/69)

I. MABs

Harrison will *not* receive marks for MABs. He will earn Up Late (to 10:00 p.m.) privilege by doing 10 to 11 of the following MABs recorded on the Daily Checklist.

1. Bed Made
2. Room Neat
3. Hair Combed (Breakfast)
4. Dress Neatly (Breakfast)
5. Hands Washed (Lunch)
6. Brush Teeth (Lunch)
7. Closets and Drawers
8. Wash Hands (Dinner)
9. Brush Teeth (Dinner)
10. Shower
11. Laundry

II. ASBs (40)

ASB-1 *Being nice or talking nicely to other kids (25)*
This ASB Category is to reward Harrison for conversation, playing well with children or any other good interaction with children. Only one other child need be involved in order for Harrison to earn marks in this category.

ASB-2 *Cooperation (5)*
This ASB Category should be used to reinforce compliance to decisions or requests made by staff. (Ex: "Let's clean up the paint you've been using.")

ASB-3 *General (10)*
All other behavior not classified in ASB-1 or ASB-2 can be reinforced by this category (Ex: good interaction with staff, doing constructive activities such as homework, etc.).

III. SCHOOL (20)
Harrison will have an earning power of 20 unit marks in school. When he earns 18 to 20 or more marks he can have a free cold drink after school. This should be a *diet* drink only!

IV. PUNISHMENT
Harrison will be on Response Cost Contingency with a mark base of 2.

Individual Contingencies:

Level 600
- 604 Assault on an Adult—1 hour TO and 50 mark fine
- 610 AWOL—1 hour TO, loss of Home Visit for one week, and 50 mark fine.
- 699 Entering Cottage Office—50 mark fine

Level 700
- 706 Self Destructive Behavior—1 hour in TO
- 709 Soiling Behavior—clean up mess and 24 mark fine

V. DIET
Because of Harrison's overweight condition he will be on a *strict* diet which includes the following:

1. *One* helping of *one* starch is allowed per meal; seconds on meat and other non-fattening foods are allowed. *One* piece of toast allowed at breakfast.
2. Desserts will be special diet desserts unless gelatin is served.
3. Snacks and treats will be fresh fruit, diet drinks or some other low calorie food.
4. Harrison will not be allowed to eat any consumables except at meals, treats, snacks, parties, or special off-unit trips to eat out. Off-unit eating trips are to be as non-fattening as possible. At parties Harrison may eat *moderate* amounts of whatever is served.
5. Possession of consumables (on person, in room) or noncompliance to this diet will be considered defiance and is to be fined accordingly.

VI. HOME VISITS

All home visits *must* be arranged in advance by Harrison's parents. The cottage staff will then be notified of home visit arrangements. Home Visit Forms (which will be in my mailbox) should be given to Harrison's parents when Harrison leaves and placed in my mailbox on his return. Any 600 Level Contingencies for that week result in loss of home visit for that week. Harrison will be rewarded for good home visits by being able to go on the off-unit activity the next Monday for free.

VII. PRICES

Arts and Crafts—FREE
Baking—5
Bed Time Story—FREE (If staff feels he has earned it)
Books—FREE
Cold Drink (after school)—18 to 20 School Marks (Diet Drink)
Comics—FREE
Contingency—R.C. Base = 2
Earning Power—ASB + MAB = 40, School = 20, Total = 60 Earned
Game Room—5 per $\frac{1}{2}$ Hour
Games—FREE
Gym—Gym Free, Tramp 5 per $\frac{1}{2}$ Hour
Home Visits—35
Breakfast
Lunch—5
Dinner
Off Unit
Bowling—20
Eat Out—30
Golf—15
Horse Ride—15
Movies—20
Ride (van)—15
Skating—15
Swimming—20

Outside
Bikes—5 per ½ Hour
Cart—5
Just Outside—FREE
Skates—FREE
Walks—Free with others, 5 per walk with only staff
Party—5
Phone Calls—5 per call (limit of 2 per week)
Recovery Charge—12
Room Visit—FREE
Snacks—5 (special diet)
Special Individual
Store Unit Base 3 per unit
T.V.—5 per ½ Hour
Treats—10 (limit 1 per eve; special diet)
Up Late—10 to 11 of MAB on Check List

VIII. PHONE CALLS

Harrison will be limited to two phone calls (5 marks per call) per week which he can make at staff convenience. Please indicate on Harrison's weekly phone call record (on the wall under his name) when he places a telephone call.

IX. CRITERIA FOR PROMOTION
1. Harrison must substantially improve his staff and peer interaction.
2. Other criteria to be determined.

Appendix D 203

MARK SHEET

ID __19__ NAME __H.L.__ DATE __LEVEL II__

Total ASB Possible: Targets 1:15, 2:10, 3:10

__15__ Total School Possible   Total MAB Possible ____

ASB–1: **BEING NICE TO OTHER KIDS**   SCHOOL

ASB–2: **COOPERATION**   JOB

ASB–3: **GENERAL**   SAVINGS / ONE / FIVE / TEN

ASB–4:

STORE____ OFF UNIT____ HOME____
PAID ON FINE____   McQueen 8/8/69

[yellow]

LEVEL II PROGRAM — HARRISON L.

(Program to begin 8/16/69)

I. MABs

Harrison will not receive marks for performing MAB's. However, he can be requested to do any that staff judges he should do (such as make his bed, clean his room or take a shower).

II. ASBs (35)

ASB-1 *Being nice or talking nicely to other kids (15)*
This ASB Category is to reward good conversation, playing well with children or any other good interaction with children. Only one other child need be involved in order for Harrison to earn marks in this category.

ASB-2 *Cooperation (10)*
This ASB Category should be used to reinforce compliance to decisions or staff requests. (Ex: "Why don't you clean up your room? No, I'm sorry, but you can't go outside.")

ASB-3 *General (10)*
All other behavior not rewarded in ASB-1 or ASB-2 can be reinforced by this category (Ex: Good positive statements, doing constructive activities such as homework, etc.).

III. SCHOOL (15)

Harrison will have an earning power of 15 unit marks in school. When he earns 13 to 15 or more marks he can have a free cold drink after school. He *cannot* buy a drink if he has not earned one.

IV. JOB (5)

Harrison can earn 5 marks for cleaning up the T.V. room and Activity room before snacks. If he has gone on an off-unit activity, time after snacks may be alloted for doing his job. He should be checked by staff to see if he has cleaned up *both* rooms. Failure to complete both earns him zero marks.

V. PUNISHMENT CONTINGENCIES

Harrison will be on Response Cost with a base of 2.

Individual Contingencies

Level 600

- 604 Assault on an Adult—1 hour in TO and 50 mark fine.
- 610 AWOL—1 hour in TO, 50 mark fine, and loss of Home Visit for one week.
- 699 Entering Cottage Office—1 hour in TO and 50 mark fine.

Level 700

- 706 Self Destructive Behavior—1 hour in TO.
- 709 Soiling Behavior—Clean up mess and a 24 mark fine.

VI. DIET

Harrison will be on the following diet:

1. *One* helping of *one* starch is allowed per meal; seconds on meat and other non-fattening foods are allowed. *One* piece of toast is allowed at breakfast.
2. Desserts should be special diet desserts unless gelatin is served.
3. Snacks and treats should be fresh fruit, diet drinks, or some other low calorie food.
4. Harrison will not be allowed to eat any consumables except at meals, treats, snacks, parties or special off-unit trips to eat out. Off-unit eating trips are to be as non-fattening as possible. Harrison is not allowed to buy consumables from the store. At parties, Harrison may eat *moderate* amounts of whatever is served.
5. Possession of consumable (on person or in the room) or noncompliance to this diet will be considered defiance and is to be treated accordingly.

VII. HOME VISITS

All home visits must be arranged in advance by Harrison's parents with Harrison's coordinator. Cottage staff will will then be notified of home visit arrangements. Home Visit Forms should be given to Harrison (if he is going home alone) or to his parents before leaving on a home visit. On returning this form should also be returned to D. F.'s mailbox.

When Harrison has had a good home visit he can go on the off-unit activity the next Monday for free. Also he will receive a ticket worth 10 marks to be used toward paying on the next home visit.

VIII. PHONE CALLS

Harrison is limited to 2 free phone calls to his family per week which he can make at staff convenience. Indicate on Harrison's weekly phone call chart (on wall under "Harrison") when he places a telephone call.

Harrison can call D. F. or K. D. when the situation warrants (e.g. when he has had a very good day, is very emotionally upset).

IX. PRICES

Arts and Crafts supplies—FREE
Baking—5
Bed Time Story—FREE
Books—FREE
Cold Drink (after school)—13 to 15 School Marks—cannot buy with marks
Comics—FREE
Contingency—R.C.
Earning Power—ASB + MAB = 40
　　　　　　　　　　　School = 15
Game Room—5 per $\frac{1}{2}$ Hour
Games—FREE
Gym—FREE
Home Visits—35
Breakfast—5

Appendix D 207

Lunch—5
Dinner—5
Bowling—20
Eat Out—30
Golf—15
Horse Ride—15
Movies—20
Ride (van)—15
Skating—15
Swimming—20
Bikes—5 per ½ Hour
Cart—5
Just Outside—FREE
Skates—FREE
Walks—FREE
Thursday Party—10
Phone Calls—FREE (limit 2 per week)
Recovery Charge—11
Room Visit—FREE
Snacks—5 (special diet)
Store Unit—Base 3 per unit
T.V.—5 per ½ Hour
Treats—5

X. "GREAT DAYS"
Each day Harrison earns 57 to 60 marks and has no fines he should be given a dated star placed on his "Great Day Chart." After Harrison earns *4* "Great Days," he can go on a special off-unit activity arranged by me.

XI. FINE PAYMENT
In order to aid Harrison pay off large fine balances in a reasonable amount of time the following procedure is to be followed:
1. If Harrison has a day with 4 marks or less in fines, he can have 250 marks deducted from his fine balance in addition to any marks he has earned.
2. For each consecutive day thereafter in which he has

no more than 4 marks in fine, his fine balance can be reduced double the amount of the preceding day plus those marks earned.

(Ex: First day with 4 or less marks in fines—250 marks substracted, second consecutive day with 4 or less marks in fines 500 marks subtracted, third day, 1000.)

3. If he, however, incurs more than 4 marks in fines for a day, the next day he will begin paying as if it were his first day (e.g. if he has 4 marks or less in fines, for that day he can have only 250 marks deducted from his fine balance).

Check fine balance sheet to determine how many marks were removed the preceding day.

When Harrison has a fine balance he can spend marks earned on a "Perfect Day" on the following day.

Appendix D

MARK SHEET

ID _____ 19 _____ NAME _____ DATE **LEVEL II - PHASE II**

Total ASB Possible: Targets 1: __10__, 2: __10__, 3: __5__

__20__ Total School Possible   Total MAB Possible _____

ASB–1: **NICE TO KIDS**   SCHOOL

			5			10
			15			20
			25			30
			35			40

			5			10
			15			20
			25			30
			35			40

ASB–2: **COOPERATION**   MAB

			5			10
			15			20
			25			30
			35			40

			5			10
			15			20
			25			30
			35			40

ASB–3: **GENERAL**   SAVINGS

			5			10
			15			20
			25			30
			35			40

ONE

			5			10
			15			20

FIVE

			5			10
			15			20

ASB–4: **BEING RESPONSIBLE ABOUT ALLERGIES**

			5			10
			15			20

TEN

			5			10
			15			20
			25			30

STORE_____ OFF UNIT_____ HOME_____

PAID ON FINE_____   McQueen 8/8/69

[yellow]

LEVEL II – PHASE II PROGRAM – HARRISON L.

(Program to begin 10/6/69)

I. MABs

Harrison will *not* earn marks for performing MABs, but should be prompted when necessary. Reinforce compliance to such requests with Cooperation marks. Do not punish failure to comply, but rather use natural contingencies where appropriate.

II. ASBs

ASB-1 *Nice to Kids*

Reward appropriate interaction with any of the other kids. This would include being a good sport, helping, friendly remarks, good conversations, etc.

10 Marks spendable + Plus Points

ASB-2 *Cooperation (Accepting Decisions)*

Reward immediate compliance to prompts and/or requests, *if* Harrison does not grumble or pout while complying.

10 Marks spendable + Plus Points

ASB-3 *General*

Emphasize joining the group! Also emphasize participation!

5 Marks spendable no Plus Points

ASB-4 *Being Responsible about his Allergies*

Reward Harrison for taking his medication, watching and being cooperative about his restricted diet, taking the initiative to sit out when he begins wheezing, etc. Emphasize doing it on his own!

10 Marks spendable + Plus Points

III. SCHOOL
Harrison's school base is *20* marks. He needs *17* out of *20* for free cold drink.

VI. JOB
Harrison is responsible for straightening up the T.V. and Activity rooms *before* snacks. If both are completed, he may go to snacks. If both or one is not done, Harrison is to go to his room and remain there.

V. PARTY
Harrison must earn 40 out of 55 marks for 2 out of 3 days to earn the party.

VI. HOME VISITS
Home visits are to be arranged through D. F. and will be posted on the "Week-end Plans" chart in the office. Home Visit Forms can be found in the large notebook ("Forms") in the office. Harrison is responsible for taking and returning these forms. When he returns, put the completed forms in D. F.'s mailbox.

Be certain that Harrison takes his medication(s) with him.

When Harrison has had a good home visit, he will receive a "Free Off-Unit Ticket" *plus* a coupon worth *20* marks toward his next home visit.

VII. PHONE CALLS
- Parents: Harrison may call his home free of charge, but is limited to *two* calls per week. A chart is posted on the wall in the office to keep track of home phone calls.
- Dick: Harrison may call Dick at any time about anything. These calls are free, and should not be stopped if Harrison is up-tight about something. It is at these times that they are especially important.

VIII. GREAT DAYS
If Harrison earns 53 marks out of 55 marks, he should be given a dated star to be placed on his "Great Day" chart. Four Great Day stars earn a special off unit with Dick.

IX. PUNISHMENT CONTINGENCY
Harrison is on Response Cost with a Base = 2.
   600 Level Contingencies
      604: 50 Mark fine + 1 hour in TO.
      610: 50 Mark fine + 1 hour in TO. + loss of next Home Visit.
      699: 50 mark fine.

X. DIET
To be decided after completion of allergy tests. For the time being, let Harrison eat whatever dietary says is OK.

XI. PRICES
Arts and Crafts—FREE
Baking—FREE
Bed-Time Story—Not Available
Books—FREE
Cold Drink after School—17 to 20 School
Comics—FREE
Contingency RC base = 2
Earning Power—20 School, 35 MAB-ASB
Game Room—5 per half hour
Games—FREE
Gym—FREE
Home Visits—40
Meals: Breakfast—5
         Lunch   —5
         Dinner —5

Off Units
Outside—FREE
Party—40 to 55 for 2 out of 3 days
Phone Calls—FREE (limit of 2 calls to home with OK)
Record Player—Pay game room
Recovery Charge—11
Room Visit—Available if had a good day (free)
Snacks—Eve. job
Store Unit Base = 2
T.V. per $\frac{1}{2}$ hour—5

Appendix D

Treats—
Up Late—
Bike—FREE
Just Outside—FREE

MARK SHEET

ID ____19____ NAME ___H.L.___ DATE **LEVEL II - PHASE III**

Total ASB Possible: Targets 1:_____, 2:_____, 3:_____

__20__ Total School Possible   No Limit   Total MAB Possible _____

ASB-1: **GOOD INTERACTION W/PEERS**   SCHOOL

			5			10
			15			20
			25			30
			35			40

			5			10
			15			20
			25			30
			35			40

ASB-2: **COOPERATION W/STAFF REQUESTS**   MAB

			5			10
			15			20
			25			30
			35			40

			5			10
			15			20
			25			30
			35			40

ASB-3: **GOOD CONVERSATION W/STAFF**   SAVINGS

			5			10
			15			20
			25			30
			35			40

ONE

			5			10
			15			20

FIVE

			5			10
			15			20

ASB-4: **MANAGING HIS ALLERGIES**

			5			10
			15			20

TEN

			5			10
			15			20
			25			30

STORE_____ OFF UNIT_____ HOME_____

PAID ON FINE_____

McQueen 8/8/69

[white]

Appendix D

LEVEL II – PHASE III PROGRAM – HARRISON L.

(Program begins 11/2/69)

This program begins the "weaning phase" for Harrison. It will also serve as an experimental perishable savings system.

NOTE: Harrison will *not* have limited earning for any of his target behaviors. It is important that he earn at approximately the same level as he has been, so continue to reinforce appropriate behavior at a fairly high frequency. Please make a conscious effort to use social reinforcement *with* the marks, as we will soon be reducing mark earning and relying more on social reinforcement.

I. PREMACKS
1. Straighten T.V. and Activity Room (earns Up Late)
2. Shower or Bath (earns snacks)

II. ASBs

ASB-1 *Good Interaction with Peers*
Reinforce all good play, conversation, work, etc., with his peer group. In the group situation, use 15 minute intervals if no specific behavior is reinforced. *Unlimited Earning*

ASB-2 *Cooperation with Staff Requests*
Reinforce compliance to staff request *only* when Harrison complies *without* grumbling or arguing. *Unlimited Earning*

ASB-3 *Good Conversation with Staff*
Reinforce any good conversations about appropriate topics (e.g. school, home, likes, dislikes, etc.). *Unlimited Earning*

ASB-4 *Managing his Allergies*
Reinforce being good about taking medication (ask nurse), being cooperative about keeping his diet, showing understanding about taking care of

himself, etc. He could earn 2 or 3 marks at a meal! *Unlimited Earning*

III. SCHOOL

Harrison's school base is 20. (18 out of 20 earns a free cold drink after school).

IV. PARTY

If Harrison has paid his "rent," the party is free. Otherwise, it is contingent on good behavior for that shift.

V. HOME VISITS

Home visits will be free and will last for three days (Friday afternoon to Monday Night) beginning November 7. Home Visit Forms are located in the "Forms Book," and should be given to Harrison before he leaves.

VI. PHONE CALLS

Harrison has unlimited, free phone calls to his home, Dick, or Chip. If it is convenient for staff, place all phone calls regardless of his emotional state.

VII. PUNISHMENT

Harrison will be on Time Out, effective November 10.
NOTE: Do not tell Harrison this before the 10th!

VIII. SAVINGS AND PLUS POINT PROCEDURES
   A. Savings: All marks earned go into General Savings.
   B. Plus Points: All marks left after paying rent Friday are recorded in Plus Points Chart kept on inside cover of his cardex.

IX. RENT

Every Friday, at approximately 3:15, Harrison will pay rent. The amount will vary, but in general it will cost 45 marks per full day on-unit. (For example: Monday thru Thursday were full days so rent is $45 \times 4 = 180$ marks). When rent has been paid, *all* activities for the next week are *free!* (See "Access to Free Activities" for exceptions and below.)

In the event that Harrison does not have enough marks to

Appendix D

pay rent, he loses access to the following for the entire week:
1. Store (missed rent by less than or equal to 10)
2. Store + Game Room (missed rent by more than 10 but less than or equal to 20)
3. Store + Game Room + T.V. (missed rent by more than 20, but less than or equal to 30)
4. Store + Game Room + T.V. + off units (missed rent by more than 30)

Mary should then be informed to write at the top of Harrison's mark sheets for the next week, "No Store + ... "
All marks in excess of those used to pay rent are Plus Points, and are recorded on sheet inside cardex.

X. G-MARK STORE ACCOUNT
Every week that Harrison pays rent, he is credited with 15 units in the store. These are to be spent during that week, and unspent store units are lost. He may purchase on the Layaway Plan. A sheet will be kept in the store as a record of Harrison's balance.

XI. ACCESS TO FREE ACTIVITIES
All free activities (i.e. he paid his rent) are contingent on appropriate behavior. Any activity can be interrupted for inappropriate behavior, but with the condition that he may rejoin the group when he feels that he is ready (at least 5 minutes later).

XII. DIET
The foods to be avoided are: 1) eggs, 2) margarine, 3) corn, 4) beef (can have it once a day), 5) anything containing the above.

LEVEL III PROGRAM – HARRISON L.
(Program begins 12/8/69)

Harrison will leave on extended home visit December 18. Until he leaves, Harrison will no longer earn marks for good behavior. Please use social reinforcement frequently when it is due! Give Harrison feedback, both positive and negative, where appropriate.

PUNISHMENT

Harrison will continue with Time Out, but will serve it in his room. School Time Outs will continue as usual.

If a punishment contingency is invoked, staff should ask Harrison why he is being sent to his room (Time Out). If Harrison gives an accurate answer to this question, cut his Time Out in half (e.g. 50 minutes T.O. reduces to 25 minutes with an appropriate answer).

PRICES

All activities are free contingent on appropriate behavior. A time out prevents access to next activity offered. Use natural contingencies where appropriate.

STORE

Harrison will be allowed to spend *20* per week in the store. A record of his balance will be kept in the store.

PREMACKS

No Time Outs in School earns a free cold drink.
Less than two TO's during the day earns snacks.
Up Late contingent on shower taken.

HOME VISIT FORM
MAB CHECKLIST

DATE:

√ = Behavior Performed
O = Behavior not Performed
X = No Opportunity

                                  Friday   Saturday   Sunday

Makes bed
Room neat
Hair combed (before breakfast)
Dressed neatly (before breakfast)
Brush teeth (breakfast)
Wash hands (lunch)
Brush teeth (lunch)
Wash hands (dinner)
Brush teeth (dinner)
Shower or bath
Picks up and puts away clothes

                                                    D. F., Counselor

DAILY REPORT: H. L.

HOME VISIT FORM

DATE: DAY:

I. Was Harrison very cooperative today?   If so, please give some examples.

II. What things went well today?

III. How did you let Harrison know that he was doing well?

IV. Where did Harrison have problems this weekend?

V. What did you do about these problems?

VI. How well did Harrison handle himself with his allergies and medicines today?

VII. Is there anything "special" that you would like to say about this weekend visit?

D. F., Counselor

Appendix E

PROGRAMS FOR TWENTY-SEVEN CHILDREN

APPENDIX E gives brief descriptions of individual programs for the twenty-seven children who are not included in Chapter 7. The program descriptions are for Subjects 1, 2, 3, 4, 5, 6, 7, 8, 9, 11, 12, 13, 14, 15, 16, 17, 18, 20, 22, 23, 24, 25, 26, 27, 28, 29, and 30. More complete case records are on file in the Adler Zone Center.

The first year of the research project was used principally to develop the program and was very much a trial and error period. The work with Subjects 1 through 8 contributed to program development, instrument development, and staff training. Much of the progressive development can be seen in the programs of these children. For the initial group of eight children, the same minimum appropriate behaviors were tokened for all children. The problem of using token earning as an indication of progress was discussed in Chapters 2 and 4. The data for these first subjects demonstrates some of the difficulty encountered in using this as a dependent variable measure.

SUBJECT I

Presenting Problems

Subject 1 (T.C.) is a nine-year-old white male of average intelligence, who was referred for treatment because of behavior problems in the home and academic problems in school.

T.C.'s family consisted of his maternal grandparents, who acted as parents, and one brother. His problem behavior with them consisted of refusing to comply with their requests, such as raising the toilet seat, going to bed on time, cleaning his room. When such requests were pursued, he would react with tantruming, screaming, throwing things, and running out of the house. The grandparents recognized that they could not manage him with their present skills, and wished to place him in another environment. An additional problem in the home was continual fighting with the brother.

Teachers reported an absence of the maladaptive behavior that appeared in the home, but T.C.'s academic work was consistently poor.

Cottage and School Programs

The following guidelines governed T.C.'s earning of tokens for appropriate social behavior.

Sharing: Any sharing that involves Martha, Keith, or Curt should be reinforced every time.
Sharing with the other children should not be reinforced every time.

Helping: Any helping behavior should be reinforced every time. Staff should try to elicit more helping behavior from T.C. by giving cues, reinforcing other kids for helping when T.C. is watching, and so forth.

Participation: Staff should try to involve T.C. in more structured activities, and the length of time he spends in the activity should be shaped. Presently he should be reinforced (on the average) for every 5 to 10 minutes of good participation.

Interaction:	Interaction with Martha, Keith, and Curt should be stressed and reinforced roughly every 15 minutes. Interaction with staff alone (includes staff reading to him) should be reinforced less frequently—roughly every 30 minutes.
Constructive:	Constructive activities should be reinforced, roughly every 15 to 20 minutes.
Individual social behavior:	Shape more normal speech tone and volume, especially in request-making situations.

T.C. was admitted for treatment in February, 1968, and remained for 56 weeks. This extra four weeks on the unit was a special arrangement between Adler and the Children's Home which he entered on discharge. The home did not have a bed available.

Data

Independent Observations

COTTAGE. The relative frequency of deviant behavior on the unit at the time observations were started, weeks 14 to 19, was low (1 to 4%). During weeks 20 to 26, those immediately preceding and including the school vacation period, the percent deviant index rose to the range of 15 to 18 percent. Percent deviant index subsided during the weeks 27 to 34, stabilizing around 10 percent. There were slight increases during weeks 35 to 36 and a fair decrease down to 1 to 5 percent during the weeks 37 to 40, but the index tended to remain around 10 to 12 percent for most of the remaining time (weeks 41 to 48).

SCHOOL. The programs established to control T.C.'s school behavior were not successful in reducing his behavior lower than the 11 to 14 percent deviant range. The program seemed to lose control of the behavior for the weeks 27 to 34, but modifications seemed to be able to reverse the negative trend and reestablish stability around 11 to 14 percent, thereafter, except for a relapse during weeks 43 to 45.

The categories of deviant behavior most frequently rated for T.C. were Out of Seat (X), Inappropriate Verbalizations (V),

Negativism *(N)*, and Inattention *(I)*. The relative frequency of X and V tended to remain constant over time. The relative frequency of N tended to increase then decrease and the relative frequency of I tended to increase over time.

Token Earning

APPROPRIATE SOCIAL BEHAVIORS. The data showed a substantial increase to nearly double in ASB token earning for T.C. during his last 12 weeks on the project as compared to his token earning during all previous weeks when ASB token earning was possible.

MINIMUM APPROPRIATE BEHAVIORS. A fairly high initial performance (85% to 90%) over an extended period indicated that the behaviors were probably in T.C.'s repertoire or were very easily established. The fluctuation in performance during the twenty-third to twenty-sixth week of treatment may have indicated that the tokens were not the most crucial variable maintaining these behaviors or that some change had taken place in the environment which devalued the tokens. It was not possible to make any valid judgment on this issue.

SCHOOL. School token earning tended to vary during the first 16 weeks. Thereafter token earning declined sharply and remained at 6 per day until school closed during the twenty-second week of treatment. When school reopened on the twenty-seventh week of treatment, token earning remained low, but there was a gradual increasing trend that generally continued until the end of residence when T.C. was earning 10.5 tokens per day.

An individualized token program for the school was instituted during the thirty-fifth week of treatment and remained in effect during the remainder of the school year. This program may have contributed to the increasing trend, although many other relevant variables were operating concurrently.

SUBJECT 2

Presenting Problems

Subject 2 (H.S.) is a twelve and a half-year old black male of average intelligence, who was referred for treatment because of behavior problems at school.

Appendix E

He was not a particular behavior problem at home; he was obedient to his father and although he tended to manipulate his mother, their relationship was described as affectionate.

At school, his behavior was aggressive and uncontrollable, and his attendance was extremely sporadic. He refused to obey the teacher, who was occasionally obliged to restrain him physically from attacking other children. His interaction with his peers consisted of fighting, pushing, roughhousing, and such. Academic performance was poor. Ultimately his behavior at school led to expulsion.

Cottage and School Programs

The following guidelines governed H.S.'s earning of tokens for appropriate social behavior.

Participation: Good participation should be reinforced roughly every 30 minutes.
Special situation: When his mood is not very good but he joins the activity, then the first few minutes of good participation should be reinforced.

Helping: Besides regular kinds of helping, give helping tokens when he helps the younger kids by encouraging them to do the right thing, et cetera.

Sharing: He should receive reinforcement fairly frequently for sharing when it is with Martha and Johnny. Sharing with Curt and Keith should be reinforced less frequently and sharing with Linda, Mitch, and Tommy should not be reinforced.

Constructive: Reinforce roughly every 30 minutes.
Reading aloud to staff should be reinforced more frequently—roughly every 15 to 20 minutes.

Cooperation: If his response is not pokey or grumpy, then reinforce it right away.
The emphasis for this category is to get him to respond to requests more quickly. No cooperation tokens should be given unless he responds fairly quickly.

Individual   Reinforce for not being grumpy in the morning,
social   especially before breakfast.
behavior: Reinforce him for noninvolvement in plotting misbehavior when the other kids are engaged in this kind of behavior.

Reinforce him for carrying on good conversations, especially when he includes the whole group. The idea here is to reinforce him for being a good model.

Data

Independent Observations

COTTAGE. The data indicated a substantial reduction of deviant behavior during the last 10 weeks of treatment. The relative frequency of Cooperation *(Co)* tended to decrease. The relative frequency of Sharing *(S)* and Helping *(H)* remained the same. Behaviors classified as Interaction tended to decrease and relative frequency of Constructive *(C)* behaviors increased steadily from 11 to 37 percent.

SCHOOL. The relative frequency of deviant behavior tended to fluctuate between 22 to 34 percent over most of the period that observations were made. The observations, as reflected in the percent deviant index, do not support any claim as to improvement in school behavior. The categories of deviant behavior most frequently rated for H.S. were Out of Seat *(X)*, Nonvocal Noise *(No)*, Inappropriate Verbalization *(V)*, Negativism *(N)*, and Inattention *(I)*. Over time, there was little change in the relative frequency of any of the above mentioned categories except *I*, which increased slightly.

Token Earning

APPROPRIATE SOCIAL BEHAVIORS. The data showed a consistent gradual increase in ASB token earning (from 6 per day to 9.9 per day) over the last 28 weeks H.S. was in residence.

MINIMUM APPROPRIATE BEHAVIORS. Performance of tokened behaviors for H.S. was fairly consistent and always above 87 percent per day. Nontokened behaviors varied in performance between 80 and 90 percent, with one five-week slump to 70 percent per day. Performance was increasing at the termination of therapy.

SCHOOL. After an initial period of instability, token earning stabilized at the 8 to 9 per day range, then at 10 per day, and finally increased gradually to 11 per day.

SUBJECT 3

Presenting Problems

Subject 3 (J.A.) is an eight-year-old white male of average intelligence, who was a behavior problem both at home and at school and also was failing to make any academic progress.

Both parents worked afternoons and evenings. Neighbors reported a great deal of socially unacceptable behavior during these hours, including some stealing.

The school reported that J.A. had been a problem since grade 1, with "amoral behavior," disturbances in the classroom, and much swearing. His teacher described him as hyperactive and aggressive towards both boys and girls. He was prone to spend much of this time with older, more deviant boys.

Cottage and School Programs

The following guidelines governed J.A.'s earning of tokens for appropriate social behavior.

Cooperation:	Each isolated incidence of cooperation should be reinforced, but when he exhibits a flurry of cooperative behaviors reinforce a few with tokens and all the rest with praise.
Helping and sharing:	These behaviors need not be reinforced with tokens as frequently as is necessary with many of the kids. But if these behaviors occur in relation to Martha, Curt, or Keith, then they should be reinforced.
Participation:	J.A. should be reinforced more frequently than every half hour—more like every 15 to 20 minutes.
Interaction:	Interaction with other children, especially with Martha, Curt, and Keith should be reinforced fair-

ly frequently—roughly every 15 to 20 minutes. Specific kinds of interactions with the staff should be reinforced:
a. When he carries on a good conversation.
b. When he responds openly and honestly, especially in those situations where he is involved in a trouble-making incident and is being questioned about it.

Constructive: Can be reinforced roughly every half hour. Staff attention during the activity is an important reinforcer for him.

Individual social behavior: In those situations where staff makes demands of him, denies him some privilege or asks him to wait with a request, any response on J.A.'s part that is not inappropriate should be reinforced.

Data

Independent Observations

COTTAGE. The data showed that since the observations were begun the relative frequency of deviant behavior remained fairly stable at 3 to 9 percent.

The relative frequencies of Cooperation *(Co)* and Interaction *(I)* tended to zigzag in downward trends so that the relative frequencies in the last nine weeks of measurement were lower than those of the first nine weeks of measurement.

Constructive *(C)* behavior also tended to go up and down, but the relative frequency in the nine weeks before discharge was more than double that in early treatment.

SCHOOL. The data indicated that there was a downward trend in the relative frequency of deviant behaviors, since measurement began in week 13, from 37 percent to 12 to 16 percent at the time of discharge.

The categories of deviant behavior most frequently rated for J.A. were Out of Seat *(X)*, Nonvocal Noise *(No)*, Inappropriate Verbalization *(V)*, Negativism *(N)*, and Inattention *(I)*. The relative frequency of X, V, and N all decreased over time. The relative frequency of No and I tended to remain low and constant.

Token Earning

APPROPRIATE SOCIAL BEHAVIOR. The data show a trend to earn more ASB tokens per day over time from 5.5 to 6.7 to 7.0 to 7.7 to 8.2 to 10.8. This trend suggested a substantial increase in performance.

MINIMUM APPROPRIATE BEHAVIORS. The only block of weeks in which performance was lower than 88 percent was that comprised of weeks 27 to 29, when it dropped to 83 percent per day. Performance of nontokened behavior was initially similar to tokened behavior but declined for several weeks until after Christmas, when it rose.

SCHOOL. The data indicated that although earning did decline from weeks 8 to 22, earning recovered to a very high level upon return to school in week 29 and remained near perfect for the rest of the residence.

SUBJECT 4

Presenting Problems

Subject 4 (M.O.) is a twelve-year-old white male of "considerable intelligence." He was referred for treatment by the Juvenile Police because of thefts of money and bicycles.

At home, his constant lying and petty theft were sources of extreme provocation to his father, who would beat him severely. The child was a source of friction between his parents and a bully toward his younger siblings.

At school he did no work, fought with his peers, and engaged in frequent emotional outbursts as attention-getting devices. Although he was considered to have a poor attitude toward learning by his teachers, his academic performance was generally at grade level.

Cottage and School Programs

The various categories of behavior were reinforced roughly every 30 minutes, but the following received special emphasis and more frequent reinforcement.

General: Reinforce in those situations where he has an opportunity to, but does not, encourage misbehavior

	in the younger kids. Reinforce him more frequently for activities such as interaction, helping, sharing, whenever he includes Martha.
Individual social behavior:	Reinforce M.O. for telling straight stories without a lot of elaborations.

Data

Independent Observations

COTTAGE. The data indicated that the relative frequency of deviant behavior remained fairly stable, 3 to 9 percent, from admission to discharge. The relative frequencies of Cooperation *(Co)* and Interaction *(I)* tended to zigzag in downward trends so that the relative frequencies of the last nine weeks of measurements were lower than those of the first nine weeks. Constructive *(C)* behavior also tended to go up and down, but the relative frequency in the nine weeks before discharge was more than double the initial nine weeks.

SCHOOL. The data indicated that there was a downward trend in the relative frequency of deviant behavior since measurement began, from 37 percent to 12 to 16 percent at the time of discharge. The categories of deviant behavior most frequently rated were Out of Seat *(X)*, Nonvocal Noise *(No)*, Inappropriate Verbalization *(V)*, Negativism *(N)*, and Inattention *(I)*. The relative frequency of X, V, and N all decreased over time; No and I remained low and constant throughout.

Token Earning

APPROPRIATE SOCIAL BEHAVIORS. The data showed a trend of increased ASB token earnings per day over time. This trend suggested a substantial improvement in performance.

MINIMUM APPROPRIATE BEHAVIORS. Performance of tokened behaviors never dropped below 88 percent per day, except for a three-week period when it averaged 83 percent per day. Performance of nontokened behaviors was initially similar but showed more fluctuation.

SCHOOL. In summary, school token earning was consistently between 9.5 to 10.5 per day during most of M.O.'s residence.

Appendix E

SUBJECT 5

Presenting Problems

Subject 5 (C.N.) is a thirteen-year-old white male of average intelligence. Behavior problems existed in the home and at school prior to admission.

In the home, a great deal of aggression and harassment of the subject's younger brother took place. The parents believed that these behaviors were intended to irritate them. The child attempted to be very manipulative of his parents and other significant adults.

At school, he refused to undress during PE. He showered in his underwear and then remained in his wet clothes all day. He also would soil himself, make no attempt to clean himself up, and thus carry a terrible odor around with him.

Personally, he had open sexual interests, with a homosexual problem very evident. According to a previous psychiatric evaluation, there was a "split between his emotional and his intellectual life, with strong antagonisms towards parents and siblings." The prognosis was said to be poor, with the possibility that the child might become psychotic.

Cottage and School Programs

C.N.'s earning power was 20 ASB's per day. These were dispensed at approximately 15 to 20 minute intervals and given to him when he emitted the desired behaviors with no time delay. The 15 to 20 minute "rule" was by no means unbreakable. During the first two weeks, staff was very sensitive to C.N. and ASB earning.

When C.N. began a new phase of Level IV, the major points of emphasis in this program were social behaviors and school behavior. He returned to a contingent level in that token earning depended solely on school behavior and ASB earning. He had a base of 15 school tokens and 20 ASB tokens. MABs and jobs were divided into the following two packets, an A.M. and a P.M. packet, which determined whether or not C.N. would be able to leave for home visits:

A.M. Packet: 1. Setting up breakfast
2. 6 MABs
P.M. Packet: 1. 4 MABs
2. Straighten up TV room
3. Straighten up game room
4. Pick up dirty laundry

Missing any one of these caused him to miss the entire packet, unless there was no opportunity to achieve some item.

C.N. paid for everything except meals at adjusted rates. Generally, high-power activities were at high cost and low-power activities were at low cost. The following handout listed special problem areas and how to deal with them.

Prices

1. Meals: Free, contingent on minimum dress requirements.
2. Home: a. 5 to 6 Packets (Monday thru Friday. A.M.) plus
   b. 50 tokens per weekend (Friday thru Sunday night)
3. Level III activities: Costs will vary according to time and/or type of activity from 5 to 25 tokens. Examples would be:
   a. Motor skill activities (i.e. skating, swimming) or low power activities—5 tokens total.
   b. Rides—10 per half hour
   c. Basketball game, play, etc.—10 tokens total
   d. Bowling—15 tokens total
   e. Movie—25 tokens total (high power)
4. Store: Same prices, but only consumable. He can purchase his gum.
5. Game Room: 5 tokens per half hour, contingent on other kids being in the game room, too.
6. T.V.: 10 tokens per half hour contingent on completion of homework.
7. Other token spending activities at same prices as now.

Data

Independent Observations

COTTAGE. The data suggests that the token contingencies had control over behavior, since percent deviant remained below 5 percent as long as token contingencies were in effect but jumped to 13 percent as soon as the contingencies were removed. The rise in deviant behavior during the last two weeks, despite the new program, may have been the result of his knowledge of imminent discharge, since he was participating in a program to reorient him to his home and community during this time.

Cooperation *(C)*, Sharing *(S)*, and Helping *(H)* all tended to decrease over time. Interaction *(I)* dropped off during late summer but recovered to 37 percent and remained there until discharge. Constructive behavior *(Co)* tended to remain stable around 28 to 32 percent, except for the weeks of Level IV noncontingent when it dropped off to 20.8 percent.

SCHOOL. The percent deviant index indicated that the program lost control of C.N.'s behavior in the school starting at week 30 and never effectively recovered it.

The categories of deviant behavior most frequently rated were Inappropriate Verbalization *(V)*, Negativism *(N)*, Inattention *(I)*, and Idiosyncratic Behaviors *(IB)*. The relative frequencies of *V*, *N*, and *I* all increased over the period of weeks 30 to 47. Thereafter there was a substantial reduction in all three. The relative frequency of IB tended to increase, but it more than doubled after the new program began in week 48. Further analysis of the data indicated a substantial decline in the more obtrusive deviant behavior after the onset of the new program. It showed that the percent deviant index was kept high by increase in the relative frequency of IB behaviors that were relatively nondisruptive.

Token Earnings

APPROPRIATE SOCIAL BEHAVIORS. The data indicated that ASB token earning was generally low, less than 50 percent per day during most of the stay on Level III. Earning picked up in the last weeks on Level III and stayed up during the contingent phase of Level IV, but dropped drastically during the noncontingent phase of Level IV.

MINIMUM APPROPRIATE BEHAVIORS. Performance was consistently high at 95 to 100 percent from week 4 to 51. There was only one lapse, during weeks 33 to 35, when performance fell to 89 percent.

The data showed highly consistent performance of both tokened and nontokened behaviors throughout the period of treatment, with tokened behaviors more frequently performed.

SUBJECT 6

Presenting Problems

Subject 6 (L.B.) is a thirteen-year-old black female of normal intelligence, who was referred for treatment by her school's social worker.

L.B.'s family was only a somewhat indifferent father, although her physical needs were well provided-for. There were no major problems, although there was conflict in the community over the father's homosexuality.

Her problems in school included speaking abusively about the teacher, talking constantly in an argumentative and pointless manner, using foul language, fighting, and threatening her peers. She was considered to have some academic potential, however.

Cottage and School Programs

The following guidelines governed L.B.'s earning of tokens for appropriate social behavior.

Participation: Good participation should be reinforced roughly every 30 minutes.

Helping: In addition to regular kinds of helping, give helping tokens when she encourages younger children to do the proper thing.

Sharing: She should be given sharing tokens often when she shares with younger children. Sharing with older children should be reinforced very infrequently.

Constructive: Continue to reinforce regularly. Encourage art work and reading.

Cooperation: She should be reinforced for all positive responses to staff suggestions.

Individual social behavior:	Reinforce personal grooming, such as washing hair or personal clothing. Reinforce for noninvolvement in plotting misbehavior when the other kids are engaged in this kind of behavior. Reinforce leadership role when she is encouraging appropriate behavior of group.

Data

Independent Observations

COTTAGE. Relative frequency of deviant behavior remained at 7 to 7.5 percent from weeks 14 to 20 before decreasing gradually over weeks 21 to 24 to 0.6 percent. In week 25, the index of percent deviant behavior jumped to 14.5 percent and then dropped 9.4 percent in the three weeks before her vacation trip. From week 31 until discharge in week 45, the index tended to stay around 10 percent, with intermittent dips to as low as 3 percent. Specifically, Coorperation *(Co)*, Helping *(H)*, and Constructive *(C)* behaviors showed a tendency to decline over time. Interaction *(I)* and Sharing *(S)* remained relatively constant.

SCHOOL. The relative frequency of deviant behavior was at 20.7 percent when observations began week 14. Except for weeks 15 to 17, when the index fell to 14.2 percent, the relative frequency of deviant behavior showed a substantial increase until vacation. When school reopened in week 27, the index was at 18.3 percent. After that, there were slight dips to as low as 6 percent. The most frequently observed categories of deviant behavior were Inappropriate Verbalization *(V)*, Negativism *(N)*, and Inattention *(I)*. V declined sharply over treatment, while N and I remained relatively constant.

Token Earning

APPROPRIATE SOCIAL BEHAVIORS. From week 11 to week 28, ASB token earning tended to fluctuate wildly, between lows of 3.4 and highs of 9.4. On the whole during this period, earning tended to fall between 5.5 and 6.0 per day. After vacation (week 31), ASB token earning stabilized at 6 to 7 per day until discharge.

MINIMUM APPROPRIATE BEHAVIORS. Performance of tokened behaviors fluctuated between 86 to 93 percent per day for weeks 20 to 28. After return from her vacation in week 31, performance remained at 98 percent or better until discharge. Performance on nontokened behaviors tended to fluctuate before week 26, but thereafter declined steadily from 85 percent to 70 to 75 percent per day, until discharge.

SCHOOL. From week 9 to week 22, earning tended to zigzag between 9 and 11 per day with the lowest earning, 7.7 per day, coming in the last week of school, week 22. Since school reopened in week 27, earning remained between 11.5 to 11.7 per day, except for one lapse during weeks 34 to 36 when she earned 10.3 per day.

SUBJECT 7

Presenting Problems

Subject 7 (K.G.) is a thirteen-year-old, white male of average intelligence. He was referred for treatment because of behavior problems in the home and at school.

At home, he was reported to be restless and preoccupied with his own thoughts. There were also reports of his shooting out a neighbor's windows with a shotgun and setting a fire in a neighbor's basement. The father said that at times he felt like "pounding K. into the ground," but he functioned such that anything the child did was all right as long as the parents were informed of it. There were indications that the mother was seductive towards the child.

At school, K.G. was inattentive, did not conform to the established rules of conduct, and seemed very indifferent to being there. He tended to avoid other children on the playground and at lunch, saying that they tended to pick on and to tease him.

In a psychiatric evaluation, K.G. was described as "hostile, antisocial in behavior, devious in most relationships, psychoneurotic with schizoid trends."

Cottage and School Programs

The following guidelines governed K.G.'s earning of tokens for appropriate social behavior.

Sharing and Helping: Reinforce whenever they occur with other children. Helping and sharing with staff should be reinforced less frequently.

Interaction: Reinforce any appropriate interaction with other children (with possible exception of card playing with just Curt). Appropriate conversation is especially important to watch for. Reinforce those K.G.—staff interactions that are improvements with adults, i.e. when he uses more appropriate attention getting devices, when conversation is relevant, when he sticks to the point but does not perseverate.

Participation: Continue to reinforce roughly every half hour of good participation.

Constructive: Reinforce roughly every half hour for constructive activities, when such an activity is appropriate.
He should not receive reinforcement when he inappropriately perseveres with one certain kind of activity.

Data

Independent Observations

COTTAGE. Up to week 51, the relative frequency of deviant behavior tended to remain fairly constant at 3 to 7 percent.

Cooperation *(Co)*, Sharing *(S)*, and Helping *(H)* showed increasing trends as did Interaction *(I)*. Constructive *(C)* behavior tended to decline.

SCHOOL. After one decreasing trend, the relative frequency of deviant behavior tended to increase in the last weeks of the old program.

The observations indicated that the most frequent categories of deviant behavior were Inappropriate Verbalizations *(V)*, Inattention *(I)*, and Idiosyncratic Behaviors *(IB)*. The relative frequency of *V* tended to decrease over time, while the relative frequencies of *I* and *IB* tended to increase.

Token Earning

APPROPRIATE SOCIAL BEHAVIOR. ASB earning stayed consistently within the 6 to 7 per day range over most of the treatment period. Lower daily earnings, in the 5.3 to 5.7 per day range, occurred during and right after Christmas break, weeks 47 to 50.

MINIMUM APPROPRIATE BEHAVIORS. After his first three weeks at the cottage, weeks 22 to 24, in which performance fell between 80 to 90 percent per day, earning stabilized in the 95 to 99 percent per day range. There was only one lapse when earning dropped to 90 percent, weeks 49 to 50. From week 22 to week 40, performance of nontokened behaviors stayed in the 88 to 92 percent per day range. Thereafter, it dropped to the 82 to 85 percent per day range.

SCHOOL. School token earning remained fairly consistent at 11 per day over weeks 24 to 43, but dropped to 10 per day in the weeks just before Christmas, weeks 44 to 45. After Christmas, earning was back up to 11.6 per day, weeks 47 to 48, but it declined in the latter weeks to 11 per day.

SUBJECT 8

Presenting Problems

Subject 8 (M.C.) is a nine-year-old white female of average intelligence. She was referred for treatment as a result of the inability of her foster parents to handle her.

The child was born with abnormal genitalia. (At age two, she had a clitoridectomy.) She had unusual sexual stimulation from a foster mother and an elderly male neighbor and frequently received attention because of her abnormal genitals. This led to her learning to expose herself to receive attention from others. Intense behavior problems, including destructive actions, began at age four when a foster boy was taken into the home.

At school, M.C. was observed to have no real friends and to lack common social skills. She had very little contact with other girls, attaching herself primarily to males. Adjustment to school was a major problem as she refused to participate in activities and threw frequent temper tantrums.

Cottage and School Programs

The following guidelines governed M.C.'s earning of tokens for appropriate social behavior.

Cooperation: Every instance of cooperation need not be reinforced, but be especially sensitive to situations where she frequently balks (such as cleaning her room) and reinforce cooperative behavior in those situations more frequently.

Sharing and Helping: When M.C. shares or helps with other children she should be reinforced almost every time.

Participation: She should be reinforced for joining an activity. Then after she is participating, the nature of the activity should be taken into account when giving reinforcement.

Participation in those activities she likes and sticks with (such as Sorry) should be reinforced roughly every 30 minutes.

Participation in more demanding activities where she is likely to give up should be reinforced more frequently (roughly every 15 minutes).

Interaction: As a general guide, any positive interaction with another child should be reinforced.

Especially watch for and reinforce any effort to engage other kids in activities. (If she has tried and failed to engage the other kids, the staff might try to help get something going and reinforce the kids more often when they "include the whole group.")

All interaction with adults should be reinforced with praise, approval, etc., rather than with tokens.

Individual social behavior: She should receive tokens for tasks (structured by staff) that are aimed at her educational deficiencies.

Listening skills: Tokens can be given if she is able to retell a story that a staff has read to her (These must be stories that are unfamiliar to M.C.).
Tokens can be given if she is able to discuss a TV program she has just seen.

Data

Independent Observations

COTTAGE. The relative frequency of deviant behaivor on the unit remained 5 percent or less during the entire treatment period, except for the two weeks before Christmas break, when it rose to 14.4 percent. Helping *(H)* tended to decrease, while Cooperation *(Co)* and Sharing *(S)* tended to remain the same. The relative frequencies of Interaction *(I)* and Constructive *(C)* behaviors decreased.

SCHOOL. The relative frequency of deviant behavior in school remained about 20 to 25 percent with no substantial changes. Most frequently rated categories were Inappropriate Verbalizations *(V)*, Negativism *(N)*, Inattention *(I)*, and Idiosyncratic Behaviors *(IB)*. *V* tended to remain low and constant. *N* decreased by half. *I* and *IB* showed a slight increase.

Token Earning

APPROPRIATE SOCIAL BEHAVIORS. Over weeks 37 to 39 and weeks 42 to 48, ASB earning per day increased from 3.8 to 9.8. In the last five weeks of treatment, earning dropped off to 8.1 and 6.9 per day.

MINIMUM APPROPRIATE BEHAVIORS. Performance of tokened behaviors steadily increased from 69 percent per day in week 31 to 95 percent per day in week 53. After the first three weeks of treatment, in which performance was 68 percent per day, performance of nontokened behaviors tended to stabilize in the 80 to 84 percent per day range for the rest of the treatment period, except for intermittent increases to 88 percent and 92 percent per day.

SCHOOL. In summary, earning generally increased over time from 8.8 per day to 11 per day.

SUBJECT 9

Presenting Problems

Subject 9 (T.Q.) is an eleven-year-old white male of average intelligence, who was referred for treatment primarily because of academic and behavior problems in the school, with additional problems at home.

The school record showed poor attendance, tardiness, and a history of academic failure. Specifically, he failed to turn in or complete assignments. He was also belligerent with teachers occasionally, and was involved in daily fist fights with his peers. Many maladaptive attention-seeking behaviors were reported also.

At home, the mother had virtually no control over his behavior. T.Q. exhibited temper tantrums and swearing when the mother attempted to get him ready for school. During school hours, he spent his time roaming through the neighborhood.

Cottage and School Programs

T.Q. was admitted for treatment on February 17, 1969. His Level I program stressed social behaviors and self-help skills. The following categories of behavior were designated as targets:

Positive statements—25 marks   Self-help skills (making
Helping and sharing—10 marks   bed, cleaning room,
General—15 marks   showering, etc.) —22 marks
                                                             School marks—15 marks

Later modifications of the program consisted of changes in the number of tokens given in each category and in the elimination of the "Helping and sharing" category after Level I. He was on Level I for four weeks, on Level II-Phase I for five weeks, on Level II-Phase II for five weeks, on Level II—Phase III for 22 weeks, and on Level III for five weeks.

Data

Independent Observations

There was a steady decrease in the percentage of the observed behaviors in the school that were deviant. During the first 10 weeks of treatment, this measure varied from 18 to 52 percent, with most values falling around 30 percent. During the last 10 weeks of treatment, values varied from 0 to 14 percent (with one exceptional week of 57%). The index showed that the percentages of positive peer, staff, and group interactions in school rose in a way that directly paralleled the decline in the percentage deviant index.

The measure showing the percentage of positive peer, staff, and group interactions on the unit remained high throughout the time of treatment, dropping below 80 percent for only two of the forty-three weeks. The index showing percentage deviant behavior on the unit was highly variable, ranging from 0 to 24 percent, with the typical values falling around 10 percent.

Daily Checklist

There were no clear trends in the performance of the behaviors on the Daily Checklist during the time of treatment. It was very seldom that either the tokened or the nontokened behaviors dropped below the 60 percent level, and at times both sets of behaviors were performed at above the 90 percent level. However, there was a great deal of variability in these measures over weeks and no apparent relation between performance levels and treatment procedures.

SUBJECT 11

Presenting Problems

Subject 11 (E.C.) is a seven-year-old white female of average intelligence, who was referred for treatment because of problems in the home situation and a history of difficulties in school.

She was cared for by her maternal grandparents. Her behavior in the home was extremely disruptive and manipulative. Much of her undesirable behavior was reinforced by the grandmother, who gave in to the child's demands whenever she would tantrum. The grandparents gave superficial agreement to home treatment plans, but they would not carry them through, with the rationalization that the causes of the child's problems were in the school situation.

The school expelled E.C. in the fall of 1968, and a homebound teacher was employed as a tutor. The same sort of manipulative behavior was seen in this situation, i.e. violent objection to correction, refusals, continued efforts at conversation during work periods.

In addition, this child showed a great deal of physical aggression with her peers.

Cottage and School Programs

E.C. was admitted to the cottage on February 24, 1969. Her program stressed maturity, friendliness with peers, and avoidance of tantrums. In an effort to gain control of her tantrum behaviors, four program levels were used during the period of treatment. On the first level, the following categories of behavior were designated as targets:

Social behaviors
    Grown-up suggestions—30 marks
    Making friends—15 marks

Self-help skills
    Meal behavior—24 marks
    Hanging up clothes—5 marks
    Picking up toys—5 marks
School behavior—20 marks
Fewer than X tantrums—snacks as reinforcer

Later changes in the program mainly consisted of added reinforcements for avoidance of tantrums. For example, on Level II candy was given at two-hour intervals throughout the day for absence of tantrums. The Level I program was begun after two weeks of baseline and lasted for four weeks. Level II was in effect for six weeks, Level II—Phase II for 16 weeks, and Level II—Phase III for nine weeks, until discharge on December 18, 1969.

E.C. was originally assigned to the time-out punishment condition. After 12 weeks, she was assigned to the response-cost condition. On August 8, she was reassigned to a time-out condition. All these conditions were modified versions of the usual cottage contingencies—modified in an effort to deal with the tantrums. During the initial time-out condition, all tantrums were ignored. The response-cost condition was the same as described in the text, with the addition that an entire fine debt could be cancelled by a day without tantrums. The final time-out condition used a chair instead of the time-out room for the lesser violations.

Data

Independent Observations

As might be inferred from the above, there was equivocal success in gaining control of E.C.'s tantrum behavior on the unit. The level of deviant behavior during the first 10 weeks of treatment varied from 0 to 7.3 percent, with most values falling around 3.0 percent. During the last 10 weeks of treatment, values ranged from 0 to 8.2 percent, with most figures occurring in the middle of this range. Similar results were found for the categories of Gross Motor, Deviant; Fine Motor, Deviant; and all of the interaction categories.

The school observations are more indicative of success. Initially, during the first 10 weeks of treatment, E.C.'s level of deviant behavior ranged from 2 to 26 percent, with most values falling around 15 percent. For the last 10 weeks, values ranged from 0 to 3 percent.

Daily Checklist

An unusual trend was seen in many of the Daily Checklist behaviors. For "bed made," "room neat," and to a lesser extent with "closets and drawers neat," E.C. performed these behaviors more frequently when they were not tokened. This pattern was maintained through ABAB contingency shifts. "Appropriate table manners" showed the reverse expected trend, i.e. an increase in frequency with tokening.

SUBJECT 12

Presenting Problems

Subject 12 (V.W.) is an eight-year-old black female, who is functionally retarded. She was admitted for treatment because of behavioral problems at home and school.

V.W.'s mother could not cope with her hyperactivity, stubbornness, and rowdy behavior. The child was characterized as jealous of her siblings and would constantly tease and yell at them until they cried.

At school, her teacher found her restless and bothersome to the class. V.W. bossed her peers around and would pick at and touch others. Her attention span in the trainable mentally handicapped class, where she had been placed, was described as very short.

Cottage and School Programs

V.W. was admitted for treatment on March 17, 1969. On Level I (4/4/69 to 5/7/69), the categories of behavior designated as targets included following staff requests; table manners (posture, correct use of utensils, napkin on lap, wiping mouth, asking for "seconds," asking to have food passed, lifting food to mouth carefully); generally appropriate social behavior; MABs (make bed, dress neatly, hair combed, room neat, wash hands for lunch, brush teeth after lunch, closets and drawers, wash hands for dinner, brush teeth after dinner, shower, laundry); and school.

On Level II (5/8/69 to 6/2/69), the targets were meal behavior; peer interaction; cooperation; MABs (same as Level I); and school.

Because V.W. was functionally quite retarded, the focus of the token program was largely on minimal self-help type behaviors at Level I, whereas expectations became more complex at Level II.

V.W. was discharged June 12, 1969, after a very short stay of three months.

Data

Independent Observations

Because of V.W.'s brief stay, only eight weeks of observational data was collected on her—an interval usually not long enough to be sensitive to behavioral changes of an enduring nature. No trends could be detected from the observations in either a positive or downward direction. Perhaps this reflected the fact that the program initially focused on self-help behaviors which would not be assessed in this data. The one major exception was percent deviant in school, which was 12, 20, and 11 percent the first three weeks and dropped to 10, 5, and 4 percent the last three weeks.

Daily Checklist

Tokened MAB performance per day for the first three weeks was around 65 to 75 percent and for the final three weeks, it fluctuated from 87 to 67 to 79 percent. Taking showers was the only minimal skill both tokened and Premacked. From an initial level of performance of 71 percent the first week, there was a climb until 100 percent per day was achieved, although the final two weeks dropped to the initial level. Behaviors never tokened were constantly performed at the 90 percent level per day.

SUBJECT 13

Presenting Problems

Subject 13 (K.R.) is a twelve-year-old white male of average intelligence, who was referred for treatment because of behavioral problems at both school and home.

At home, the problems centered around his uncontrollable temper tantrums. On several occasions, he beat up his mother, threw furniture around, and tore up his own clothes. Nocturnal enuresis was another major problem.

Constant fighting at school led to his expulsion. Academically, his progress had been very slow due to conspicuous lack of motivation. Grade 4 was the last grade completed at admission.

Cottage and School Programs

K.R. was admitted for treatment on March 24, 1969.

On Level I (4/19/69 to 5/14/69), the categories of behavior designated as targets included sportsmanship; understanding; MABs (dress neat, comb hair, room neat, hands-lunch, teeth-lunch, closets and drawers, hands-dinner, teeth-dinner, shower, laundry); and school.

On Level II (5/15/69 to 8/14/69), the targets were sportsmanship; conversation (soft talk at meals); MABs (same as Level I); and school.

On Level III (8/15 to discharge), the targets were friend-making behaviors; and school.

At Level III, MABs ceased to be either tokened or Premacked. The backup for appropriate social behavior on Levels I and II was the privilege of spending time off unit.

K.R. was discharged Sept. 22, 1969.

Data

Independent Observations

In general, observations showed a deterioration or lack of change in performance in virtually all categories during his stay on the unit. Percent deviant behavior averaged around 2 percent during his initial five weeks on the unit, but fluctuated from 4 to 14 percent during the five weeks before discharge. In school, percent deviant was high almost throughout, on several occasions in the 30 to 40 percent level. The initial and final levels were approximately 12 percent. The only category in which positive improvement was shown was unit positive gross motor behavior, which increased steadily from an initial 22 percent to a final 67 percent level.

Daily Checklist

Performance of tokened behaviors was usually around the 85 to 95 percent per day level; however, when the tokens were removed (5/14/69), performance deteriorated after a few weeks to the 60 to 70 percent level. Performance of behaviors never tokened showed a slight decrease over time from the 85 to 95 percent level to the 80 to 90 percent level. This decrease corresponded roughly to the deterioration that occurred when tokens were removed from the self-help behaviors initially receiving them.

SUBJECT 14

Presenting Problems

Subject 14 (D.H.) is a twelve-year-old white male of dull-normal intelligence, who was referred for treatment because of problems in the home, school and community.

At the time of referral D.H. was not in school, since he had been suspended for unacceptable behavior. He reportedly engaged in negative, attention-seeking behaviors, such as shooting rubber bands, poking, and kicking at others. He reportedly was defiant of any rules made in the home, particularly those made by his mother. He frequently stayed out late at night and occasionally stayed out all night. At age 10, D.H. was arrested for the first time for stealing money from a parking meter. Since that time, he has been in difficulties with the authorities for stealing a check, vandalizing a ladies restroom, stealing dramamine from a drug store and being an accomplice in the theft of a car.

Cottage and School Programs

During a three week Orientation Level on the cottage, D.H. was observed to get angry and to tantrum in response to any restrictions that prevented his getting what he wanted. At times he exhibited immature behaviors, such as breaking into tears over minor disappointments and clinging onto staff members.

The following categories of behavior were designated as targets:

> Accepting decisions—15 marks
> General—15 marks
> Self-care behaviors: neatly dressed; hair combed; room neat; washing hands, lunch and dinner; closets and drawers neat; taking a shower; and putting out his laundry—15 marks
> School marks—18 marks

Later modification of the program consisted of marks being given for any generally good behavior. Special procedures were that all reinforcers, other than the store, were free for D.H. as long as his behavior was appropriate. One special condition was set up regarding off-unit activities. He was allowed to participate in an off-unit activity as long as he had not been in Time Out more than once during the day.

Home Program

D.H.'s family was not regarded as a suitable placement for D.H. Since he was a ward of the court, plans were made to place him in a boy's home. Cottage personnel worked with the staff of boys' home in order to insure that D.H. would be able to make the transition from Adler.

Data

Independent Observations

During D.H.'s Level 1 program, deviant behavior was observed to decrease and positive responses increased on the unit; later after being placed on response cost, the percent of deviant behavior was quite variable and there was a slight decrease in the percent of positive interactions. The percent of positive peer interactions was variable but generally increased during his stay in Adler. In the beginning weeks of D.H.'s school program, both positive and deviant behavior were variable; later there was a considerable increase in the percentage of positive behaviors. Behaviors that were rated positive included such things as being on task, and obeying instructions from the teacher.

Daily Checklist

Those MAB behaviors that were never given concrete reinforcement continued to be performed at approximately the same rate throughout D.H.'s stay. Those self-care behaviors that were tokened showed a considerable increase over the level of performance during the orientation period.

SUBJECT 15

Presenting Problems

Subject 15 (M.D.) is a thirteen-year-old black male of normal intelligence, who was referred to Adler because of disruptive, defiant, bizarre behavior at school and belligerent, defiant behavior at home. M.D.'s mother is a white woman who has been diagnosed as a chronic schizophrenic.

Cottage and School Programs

M.D.'s interaction during the first three weeks on the cottage was very poor. When he did react with others, he was loud, silly, told many hard-to-believe tales, and made many impossible threats. M.D.'s responses were often irrelevant and his reasoning paranoid.

The general goals of M.D.'s program were to increase his interest in and success with other people and to decrease negative statements and paranoid, fantasy behavior. The following four categories of social behavior were defined as targets:

    Joining groups   Positive statements—
    (participation) —15 marks   15 marks
    Helping—10 marks   General—15 marks

The "General" category was used to reinforce any good behavior displaying a realistic perception of a situation in daily living, e.g. saying "I couldn't have dessert because I didn't eat dinner" rather than "I couldn't have dessert because staff hate my color." Many self-care behaviors were Premacked. For example, if he washed his hands before meals and brushed his teeth after meals, then he earned a snack in the evening. Later, only two targets were designated:

    Self-confidence—10 marks   General—15 marks

The "Self-confidence" category was used to reinforce behaviors leading to M.D.'s being able to conduct himself and to manage his affairs with confidence in the community. In the final stages of his program his target behaviors were designated as follows: tell it as it is, playing it straight, General, and serious basketball. "Serious basketball" was used to reinforce M.D. for practicing for the basketball team at the junior high school.

In the Adler school, M.D. was given 15 spendable marks a day for academic and social behavior. Later marks earned in public school performance earned him special meals and opportunity to attend the weekly cottage party. Free time in the game room was earned by having a perfect school day.

One of M.D.'s public school teachers and his family became interested in taking M.D. as a foster child. Adler staff and the caseworker from the Department of Children and Family Services met with this family before and after discharge.

Data

Independent Observations

The percentage of positive interactions and positive verbalizations showed an overall increase while at Adler. The percentage of deviant behavior showed a marked decrease over the Orientation Level. In school, the percentage of positive interactions showed an upward trend from an initial 50 to 60 percent level. The percentage of deviant behavior in school decreased from a 35 to 40 percent level to a 0 to 10 percent level.

Daily Checklist

Those behaviors that were not felt to require a systematic contingency were performed at a higher level after M.D.'s Level I program began than at Orientation Level and this high level of performance continued. Staying up late proved to be an effective motivation for showering, putting out laundry and getting to bed on time.

SUBJECT 16

Presenting Problems

Subject 16 (C.G.) is a thirteen-year-old white female of superior intelligence (Stanford Binet I.Q. score: 152). She was referred for treatment because of social isolation and nonperformance of self-help skills, both at home and in the school.

Her parents were divorced when she was five years old. From that time until the mother's recent remarriage, C.G. had been able to control and manipulate the mother. She resisted the stepfather's attempts to set limits verbally and physically. She had withdrawn more and more from her family since the mother's remarriage, and had threatened to run away and become a hippie. Towards a younger brother, she was either ignoring or highly authoritarian.

At school she would make shocking or repulsive statements, would stare or grimace at others, and on occasions when she thought she was being treated unfairly, she would have hysterical outbursts. She would also force her way into adult conversations.

Most of her time, though, would be spent reading or daydreaming, isolating herself from the other children. She was making little academic progress, relative to her apparent capacity.

Personally, she was very obese, with hair and dress unkempt. Her interaction style was a kind of pseudointellectualism, which was somewhat inconsistent with her emotional immaturity.

Cottage and School Programs

C.G. was admitted for treatment on April 9, 1969. Her program stressed interaction with others (nonisolation) and improvement of personal appearance. On her Level I program, the following categories of behavior were designated as targets:

Being friendly—20 marks General—10 marks
Joining large groups—10 marks School behavior—20 marks

Later modifications of her program added categories for "Exercises" and "Looking Nice." These behaviors were maintained primarily through social reinforcers and Premack contingencies.

Data

Independent Observations

At the school, there was a clear decrease in the percentage of deviant behavior observed. During the first 10 weeks of treatment (weeks 64 to 73), the percentage deviant index ranged from 0 to 21.9 percent, with most values around 10 percent. For the last 14 weeks of treatment, this index ranged from 0 to 4.0 percent, with all but three weeks at zero percent. A corresponding decrease was seen in the measure reflecting percentage of deviant verbalization in school.

On the unit, there was no clear increase or decrease over time in any category.

Daily Checklist

During the time of treatment, there were positive changes in the categories of hair combed, shower, laundry, in bed on time, and dressed neat. All were associated with Premack contingencies. More erratic were the changes in the categories of closets and drawers, room neat, brush teeth, bed made, and wash hands. Values for these latter categories varied from 0 to 100 percent and showed no consistent pattern.

SUBJECT 17

Presenting Problems

Subject 17 (T.K.) is a seven-year-old white female of average intelligence, who was referred for treatment because of behavioral problems at home.

She was born with a congenital intestinal defect called colostomy, which rendered excretory functioning very difficult and required that she have a bag attached to her person for that purpose. The child's mother developed hostility toward her because of the extra care she required and the financial costs incurred, which forced the mother to work at night (T.K. has had several operations).

At school, her progress was only a little less than grade level. Her behavior was generally quiet and withdrawn, except for occasional temper tantrums. A major problem was that she was avoided both at home and at school because of her colostomy, which caused her to have a foul odor.

Cottage and School Programs

T.K. was admitted to the treatment program April 30, 1969.

On Level I (5/8/69 to 6/22/69), the categories of behavior designed as targets included interaction with peers, self; initiated activity; being prompt; general (cooperation, helping, sharing with others); MABs (colostomy, bedmaking, room neat, shower, pants off at night); and school.

On Level II (6/23/69 to 8/21/69), the targets were interaction with peers; general (cooperation, being prompt, constructive activity); MABs (bag checks, room neat, bedmaking); and school.

T.K.'s colostomy necessitated teaching self-help skills in that area, including controlling leakage of her bag and cleaning up any accidents that did occur.

She was discharged August 21, 1969.

Data

Independent Observations

Positive interaction with peers on the unit, a major target behavior, showed an upward trend from an initial 5 to 8 percent level to a final 12 to 21 percent level for the first and last three weeks. Negative verbalizations also showed an increase. In school, positive interaction with self and objects, positive gross and fine motor behavior, and negative verbalizations also showed increases.

In general, percent deviant behavior in both school and unit, initially less than the 5 percent the first three weeks of her stay, increased in both cases to near the 10 percent level in the three weeks prior to discharge.

Daily Checklist

Performance of tokened self-help behaviors (bed made, room neat, shower) was poor throughout her stay and actually deteriorated over time to where she was only performing at a 60 percent and 44 percent level per day the last two weeks. Nontokened behaviors were performed at a somewhat higher, but still rather low level (usually 65 to 80% level) throughout. Doing laundry, first not tokened and then Premacked, showed an increase from a 33 percent performance level the first two weeks to a 100 percent level for the last two weeks.

SUBJECT 18

Presenting Problems

Subject 18 (L.B.) is an eight-year-old white male, who was referred for treatment because of problems at home and at school.

His family consists of a mother and stepfather. L.B.'s behavior in the home was disruptive and unacceptable to the parents, particularly the stepfather. Specifically, L.B. would speak loudly and out of turn, lie, try to sabotage the stepfather's attempts at discipline, and act in a way disrespectful of authority.

In school, he tended to talk loudly all the time, forget to raise his hand, and to act defiant or "smart." He also seemed to be very restless and excitable. Demands for teachers' attention were excessive. On the positive side, his motivation for academic achievement is very high.

He seemed like a very unhappy child, with some lack of self-control. He did not seem to have adequate outlets for emotion except motorically. He also reported his perception that the parents, particularly the stepfather, wanted to get rid of him.

Cottage and School Programs

L.B. was admitted to the program on June 8, 1969.

General goals were a school program that would allow him to reach his intellectual potential; inner discipline and controls; a good relationship with one person; and limits on objectionable behavior (defiance, talking out, etc.).

The Level I program began two weeks after admission, and the following categories of behavior were designated as targets:

>   Cooperation—15 marks
>   Playing with kids—15 marks
>   General (soft talking when appropriate, meal behavior) —10 marks
>   Job—5 marks

The job consisted of making his bed in the morning, keeping his room neat, and emptying his waste basket. There were no school marks given. The Level II program, which ran from July 22 to August 15, 1969, differed only in that "soft talk" was made a category by itself, marks were given for PE performance, and an evening job was added. Modifications were made to Level II on August 16. These included making the special breakfast contingent upon the performance of the evening job. Mark-earning power was reduced from 65 to 20. The Level III program (September 19-25, 1969) was based entirely on Premack contingencies. Blocks of time free from time outs led to special breakfast, lunch, cold drink after school, dinner and snacks in the evening, provided the jobs were also done. He was discharged on September 25, 1969.

Data

Independent Observations

There were no clear trends in the percentage of deviant behavior observed during the time of treatment, either on the unit or in school. Weekly values for this measure varied from 3.5 to 29.0 percent, with figures typically in the 8 to 12 percent range. There were encouraging changes in the percentages of desirable verbalizations that were observed, both on unit and at school. During the time of treatment, these figures rose from around 15 percent to around 30 percent in the school and from about 25 percent to around 40 percent on the unit.

Daily Checklist

The behaviors on the Daily Checklist that were attached to reinforcing contingencies occurred with consistently greater frequency than those without contingencies. Performance of both reinforced and nonreinforced behaviors was initially low, but increased during treatment, with several "perfect weeks" occurring for reinforced behaviors toward the end of treatment.

SUBJECT 20

Presenting Problems

Subject 20 (D.S.) is a twelve-year-old white female of dull-normal intelligence with a history of epilepsy, who was referred for treatment because of problems in both the home and school.

At the time of admission, D.S. was attending school only part-day because of her frequent assaults on other children and threats toward teachers. At home she had difficulty relating to her three sisters. It was reported that there were few times when they could be together without a fight or argument starting.

Cottage and School Programs

During the three-week Orientation Level, D.S. had high frequencies of teasing, provoking and hitting her peers. She was also observed to steal things from others.

On Level I, the categories of behavior designated as targets included: interaction; cooperation; helping; positive statements; MABs (taking a shower, and putting out laundry); and school.

On Level II, the targets were: being friendly; cooperation; independence; communicating with staff; MABs (making bed, room neat, and showering); and school.

On Level II-Phase II, the targets were: independence and self-initiative; being friendly; general; MABs (making bed, room neat and showering); and school marks were given for performance in the public school.

After the Orientation Level, D.S. made almost weekly home visits. Her parents met weekly with D.S.'s Extramural Case Coordinator to discuss D.S.'s program. The parents cooperated with the program, recording incidents of punishable behavior and giving points for good behavior. These meetings with parents continued after discharge.

Data

Independent Observations

The observer data indicates a definite decrease in the incidence of deviant behavior after Orientation Level. This decrease was maintained throughout her stay at Adler. Positive interactions were stressed throughout her program and data related to interactions indicate steady improvement. In general, observer ratings of deviant behavior in the classroom does not indicate much change. The most gain seem to be made after she began to attend public school part time.

Daily Checklist

Several behaviors on the Daily Checklist had special contingencies. The results of these contingencies were not consistent, and overall it cannot be said that there was any change in this behavior.

SUBJECT 22

Presenting Problems

Subject 22 (B.G.) is a ten-year-old white male of normal intelligence, who was referred for treatment because of behavior problems at school.

His parents were described as over-involved and reacting with alarm to his school problems. B.G. was characterized as nervous, lacking in self-confidence, vacillating between passivity, impertinency, and tantruming. Frequent behaviors included daydreaming and crying.

At school, he was quick to get mad and blow up. Academically, he was duplexic, constantly near failing, and in fact had to repeat first grade.

Cottage and School Programs

B.G. was admitted July 17, 1969, and discharged October 31, 1969. Thus his total stay in the cottage was only three and a half months.

On Level I (8/4/69 to 9/29/69), the categories of behavior designated as targets included working on reading; generally appropriate social behavior; MABs (bed made, room neat, closet and drawers); and school.

On Level II (9/30/69 to 10/31/69), the targets were working on reading; growing up; and general (especially self-confidence and enthusiasm).

On Level II, B.G. was given the job of emptying waste baskets, which was Premacked using snacks as a reinforcer.

B.G. was on baseline from 7/17 to 8/3 and response-cost punishment condition from 8/4 to discharge. In neither condition was his frequency of deviant behavior usually in excess of zero per day.

Data

Independent Observations

Percent deviant behavior remained low throughout his stay, never exceeding 15 percent on the unit and 5 percent at school. The data in specific categories showed no consistent trends in either the positive or negative categories. There was a tendency for week-to-week fluctuations of considerable magnitude in many categories.

Daily Checklist

Performance of nontokened behaviors remained between 85 percent and 95 percent until a drop in 12 percent at discharge. Self-help skills that initially were not tokened (bed made, room neat, closets and drawers) showed a dramatic increase in percent performance per day when tokened, from a low of 40 percent to a level of 100 percent for six of the seven weeks before discharge.

SUBJECT 23

Presenting Problems

Subject 23 (R.S.) is an eleven-year-old black male of low average intelligence, who was referred for treatment because of predelinquent behavior.

He ran away from home on several occasions, complaining of whipping and bad conditions there. His mother is frequently very harsh in her disciplinary techniques, and plans to have guardianship taken over by the Department of Children and Family Services were currently being instituted because of parental neglect at the time of admission.

Personally, R.S. was passive, quiet, and withdrawn. His academic performance at admission was on the first-grade level in most subjects, including reading. Neighborhood predelinquent behavior included stealing bikes, taking small objects from stores, and associating with other boys with legal records.

Cottage and School Programs

R.S. was admitted to the cottage September 15, 1969.
On Level I (10/8/69 to 11/9/69), the categories of behavior designated as targets included cooperation, interaction, and generally appropriate behavior.

On Level II (11/10 to 12/18/69), the target behaviors were cooperation, interaction, generally appropriate behavior, and conversation.

On Level II-Phase II (12/19 to end of project), the target behaviors were cooperation, interaction, reading, and clear speech.

Beginning with Level II, he was given the job of emptying

wastebaskets in the cottage bedrooms. No tokens were received for this duty; a snack was used as a reinforcer instead.

Data

Independent Observations

Percent deviant on the unit at admission was rather low and remained that way throughout treatment. It never exceeded 12 percent for any one week and generally tended to be around the 2 to 5 percent level. Although at no period was there ever a significant amount of negative interaction with peers, groups, or staff, the frequency of total positive interaction declined somewhat over time. Interaction with self and objects remained consistently high and often exceeded the sum of the other three interaction dimensions combined.

Percent deviant at school fluctuated from 0 to 17 percent, but generally was between the 2 to 6 percent level. Positive interaction with the group increased dramatically over time. Positive verbalization showed a steadily increasing trend.

Daily Checklist

As R.S.'s self-help skills were satisfactory, none were ever tokened. Performance, however, was never perfect for any given week and usually was within the 70 to 85 percent range.

SUBJECT 24

Presenting Problems

Subject 24 (C.B.) is a thirteen-year-old white, functionally retarded female, who was referred for treatment because of behavior problems in both the home and school situations.

Her family consists of her mother, stepfather, and three younger siblings. Her behavior in the home was described as restless, disruptive, disobedient, and uncooperative. She reportedly took hours to complete tasks and was constantly seeking attention.

In school, she had been in an educable mentally handicapped classroom where she was functioning academically on the second-grade level. Her school attendance had been erratic. In the classroom, she was described as talking constantly, using abusive language, being hyperactive, and distracting others. She had not developed satisfactory peer relations and was characterized as being overly aggressive towards her peers, especially the boys.

Cottage and School Programs

C.B. was admitted for treatment on September 22, 1969.

The emphasis of her program was on developing compliance with adult requests, appropriate conversation, and more ladylike behavior.

On Level I, the following categories of behavior were designated as targets:

Compliance—15 marks   MABs—10 marks
Conversation—15 marks   School—20 marks
Generally appropriate behavior—15 marks

On Level II, the targets were the same as Level I, with the exception that "Ladylike behaviors" were added to the social behaviors category.

She was on the Level I program for eight weeks, and at the end of the project, she had been on her Level II program for 20 weeks. C.B. was initially assigned to the time-out punishment condition, which was in effect for 14 weeks. After a second baseline period of two weeks, she was changed to response cost and experienced this punishment condition for twelve weeks.

Data

Independent Observations

The data indicates an immediate and fairly consistent reduction in the percentage of deviant behavior observed on the unit. The one exception to this pattern was a fairly high rate of deviant behavior (38.1%) during the first week of the punishment baseline. The mean level of deviant behavior during orientation was 26.7 percent, while the mean level during the last 10 weeks of treatment was 10.5 percent. Deviant behavior in school showed considerable variability when the program first started, but showed some stability at a lower level in the last 10 weeks. Mean level of deviant behavior in the school during orientation was 17.3 percent, while the mean for the last 10 weeks was 5.2 percent.

Negative peer interactions observed on the unit showed a considerable decrease. The mean level of negative peer interactions during orientation was 16.3 percent, while the mean level for the last 10 weeks was 4.5 percent. The one week that showed an exception to this pattern was the first week of punishment baseline, when the observed level of negative peer interaction was 25.5 percent. Negative peer interactions in school initially increased (the mean level during orientation was a very low 1.7%), but in the last 12 weeks, has decreased to a level slightly below that during orientation (mean of 1.1%).

Observations on the unit indicated an immediate and consistent decrease in negative verbalizations. The mean level during orientation was 18.2 percent, compared to 7.9 percent during the last 10 weeks of treatment. The only exception to this consistent pattern of reduction was the first week of the punishment baseline when the level of negative verbalizations was 33.5 percent. Along with the decrease in negative verbalizations on the unit, there was also an increase in the level of positive verbalizations.

The amount of time during which she was observed to be engaged in positive interaction with people generally increased over that shown during orientation, when the mean level of positive interaction with people was 40.5 percent. During the last 10 weeks of treatment, the mean level was 54.1 percent. The mean for the last 10 weeks of treatment was 87.4 percent, whereas the mean during orientation was 64.2 percent.

The percentage of positive interactions with adults observed in both the school and on the unit were considerably increased over orientation. The mean level of positive interactions with adults during orientation was 65.1 percent on the unit and 83.0 percent in school. During the last 10 weeks of treatment, the mean level for the unit was 89.7 percent and for the school was 94.2 percent.

Appendix E

SUBJECT 25

Presenting Problems

Subject 25 (P.M.) is a twelve-year-old white female, who is retarded due to cerebral palsy. She is the twin sister of Subject 26. P.M. obtained an I.Q. score of 54 on a 1964 administration of the Stanford-Binet, and a score of 45 on a 1966 administration of the Lester Performance Scale. She was referred for treatment in order to learn specific self-help skills and greater independence in general.

At home, she would consistently test her parents' limits. The loudness of her voice was often unnecessarily high, and she would not practice certain basic self-care skills, such as washing her own hair and taking baths, without close supervision. Also, she was very jealous of her sister's (Subject 26) superior physical skills and greater independence. She would not tolerate others touching her, and would assault any strangers who touched her.

Her school record showed that she possessed certain very basic academic skills, i.e. she knew her colors, could count to three, and could print with extreme difficulty. She had a good relationship with her teacher, but was absent much. Though generally isolative from her peers, there was one instance of her having initiated a peer relationship.

Cottage and School Programs

She was admitted for treatment on October 6, 1969. The goals of the cottage program were to develop the ability to be independent in some activities; the ability to express anger and aggression without hitting; greater speaking ability; self-care skills; improved facility at walking; improved relationship with her sister; and acceptance of the home structure.

On Level I, the following categories of behavior were designated as targets:

Mealtime behavior—20 marks	General—10 marks
Conversation—15 marks	School behavior—30 marks
Being nice to sister—12 marks	

On Level II, the targets were as follows:

Being alert at mealtime—12 marks Bedmaking and bathing
Being alert—20 marks   —8 marks
Playing—10 marks   School—15 marks

Subject 25 was placed on the time-out punishment contingency from November to February. After a return to baseline for two weeks, she was placed on the response-cost contingency.

Data

Independent Observations

On the unit, there was a clear increase in the amount of positive interactions with the cottage staff. During the first five weeks of treatment, the index measuring this behavior varied from 1.5 percent to 10.9 percent; for the last five weeks on the project, these figures ranged from 10.3 to 19.1 percent. Other measures of behavior on the unit and in the school showed no clear trends.

Daily Checklist

There was a steady increase in performance of the behaviors on the Daily Checklist. During the first five weeks of treatment, aggregate performance consistently fell at about the 75 percent level, with relatively little variation. In latter weeks, this index climbed to the 92 percent level on four occasions, but also with considerably more variation from week to week. The two check list behaviors that had token contingencies rose in frequency, from the 42 percent level to a consistent 100 percent performance.

SUBJECT 26

Presenting Problems

Subject 26 (P.M.) is a twelve-year-old white female, who is retarded due to cerebral palsy. She is the twin sister of Subject 25. Subject 26 obtained an I.Q. score of 48 on a 1969 administration of the Wechsler Intelligence Scale for Children. She was referred for treatment in order to learn specific self-help and social skills.

In the home, she would argue a great deal with the mother when she tried to set limits, but eventually she would meet requirements. One of the child's main problems was in getting along with her sister, toward whom she was very antagonistic and aggressive. She seemed to be somewhat jealous of the sister's ability to attract adult attention. A third sister was becoming jealous of both twins because of the time the parents had to spend with them.

In 1968, she was transferred to a special class for the socially maladjusted because of aggressive behavior in a class for the emotionally and mentally handicapped. Here she was at first aggressive toward the teacher, but then later was able to form an emotional relationship with her. Upon admission, her reading was at the grade-one level. She reported enjoying reading, but did not like arithmetic. She was able to count to 100 and to write numbers.

Cottage and School Programs

She was admitted for treatment on October 6, 1969. Treatment goals were to teach her to tolerate frustration without becoming aggressive; to relate to peers; to speak in a way that was more easily understood; to tend to her personal cleanliness and grooming; to improve her ability to walk; to get along with her sister; and to accept the home structure.

Her Level I program included the following categories of behavior as targets:

Good conversation—15 marks
Mealtime behavior—20 marks
Ignoring sister when she is talking to herself—5 marks
Cooperation with staff—15 marks
Being nice to sister—10 marks

On Level I—Phase II, the targets were as follows:

Eye contact and clear speech—20 marks
Interaction—15 marks
Cooperation—10 marks
General—5 marks

On Level II, the targets were as follows:

Being responsible—20 marks   Clear speech—10 marks
Sharing—15 marks   General—5 marks
Interaction—15 marks

This child was placed on the time-out punishment condition.

Data

Independent Observations

On the unit, there was wide variability and no clear pattern in the percentage deviant index. There was a slight positive trend in the percentage of all verbalizations that were positive. Observers recorded a great increase in the extent to which staff members reinforced Subject 26 during the last seven weeks of treatment. This may be an indication of desirable, but nonmeasured, behavior changes.

Daily Checklist

There was a steady increase in the extent to which nontokened Daily Checklist behaviors were performed. During the time of treatment, performance levels for these behaviors increased from about 70 percent to around 90 percent. There was much more variability in the check list behaviors that were connected with token contingencies, and thus no clear trend of improvement emerged.

SUBJECT 27

Presenting Problems

Subject 27 (B.R.) is an eight-year-old white male of normal intelligence, who was referred for treatment because of problems in both the home and school.

Prior to admission to the treatment program, observations were made of B.R.'s classroom behavior. He was observed to emit such behaviors as walking around the classroom, taking objects out of desk and off of shelves, playing with toys, speaking to other children or speaking to teacher out of turn. B.R. was observed to emit these behaviors 83 percent of the time that he was observed. The parents reported that he frequently becomes angry with his mother and at these times will verbally attack her, destroy things which she values, throw something at her or assault her physically.

Cottage and School Programs

During the three week Orientation Level, B.R. was observed to emit an average of 46 punishable behaviors per day, with particularly high frequencies of behaviors that fall into the categories labeled verbal abuse, defiance, assault, and threatening others.

On Level I, appropriate mealtime behavior, positive interactions with younger children, and "generally pleasant behavior" were targets. B. R. received marks for the performance of all the self-care behaviors listed on the Daily Checklist, with the exception of items related to behavior at meals. B.R. was able to earn a total of 70 spendable marks for his performance and behavior in school. These marks were given for such behaviors as being in seat and paying attention. He was allowed to earn approximately one mark for every three minutes he was in class. He remained on his Level I program for sixteen weeks.

On Level II the targets in B.R.'s program were minding mother and father, interactions with other kids, positive discussion with Intramural Counselor, and meal behavior. Ten marks were available on this program to reinforce self-care behaviors that were labeled "Just like home behaviors." These behaviors were making bed, picking up room, dressing neatly, and so forth. B.R. began attending the public school. A system was set up where by he earned school marks for appropriate school behavior in the public school.

Home Program

During and following B.R.'s stay at Adler, work was done with the parents by a member of the Research Project Staff and by the Psychological Clinic at the University of Illinois. The parents were taught the basic principles of contingency management as outlined in *Living With Children*.

Data

Independent Observations

COTTAGE. The percentage of deviant behavior decreased as soon as his Level I program began and remained for thirteen weeks when there was a great increase. Another increase occurred during the week that time-out procedure were instituted. After that the rate of deviant behavior again declined. The percentage of positive peer interactions followed the pattern described above: less deviant behavior more positive interactions.

SCHOOL. There was considerable variability in the percent of deviant behavior in school. B.R. did demonstrate that his behavior could improve and there was a downward trend at the end of his stay at Adler.

Daily Checklist

All behaviors appearing on the Daily Checklist were at sometime followed by a systematic contingency period. There was a general upward trend in all of these behaviors. Mealtime behavior is of particular interest since it was identified as a target on both Level I and Level II programs. As soon as the Level I program began, there was a dramatic increase in his performance of appropriate mealtime behavior. This increase was generally maintained throughout his treatment program.

SUBJECT 28

Presenting Problems

Subject 28 (T.C.) is an eight-year-old white male of low average intelligence, who was referred for treatment because of frequent running away from home.

T.C.'s family was characterized as financially, educationally, and socially deprived. There was inadequate training, structure, and physical care for the children. The child began running away while in grade one, often physically endangering himself in the process. Other deviant behaviors in the neighborhood included shoplifting, street-begging, and stealing bicycles.

At school he was restless, easily distracted, and unable to get along with his peers. His record included excessive absences and running away from school. Academically, he was classified as a slow learner with speech and language problems.

Cottage and School Programs

T.C. was admitted December 1, 1969. On Level I (12/19/69 to 3/11/70), the categories of behavior designated as targets were positive interaction with younger kids; grownup suggestions; courtesy (especially toward property); and minimal acceptable behaviors (bed, room neat, closets and drawers, dressed neat, meals).

On Level II (3/12/70 to end of project), the targets included interaction, grownup suggestions, asking permission and returning things, responsibility, and MABs.

Maximum number of marks possible was 81 during Level I and 74 during Level II. During the latter level, T.C. was given the job of cleaning the study hall at evening. If the job was done satisfactorily all week, the reward was a toy.

Data

Independent Observations

Total percent deviant behavior on the unit showed considerable fluctuation from 0 to a high of almost 30 percent. During the last six weeks recorded, however, it did not exceed 8 percent. No clear trends emerged in any of the specific categories. In school, percent deviant showed a steady increase from a low initial level. Interactions with peers and staff at school, both positive and negative, showed a definite increase over orientation.

Daily Checklist

On Level I, the self-help behaviors that were both tokened and Premacked included bed made, room neat, closets and drawers, dressed neatly, and brush teeth after all meals. Good manners and good social behavior during meals received tokens only. Showers, laundry, and being in room on time were Premacked. On Level II, meal-behavior manners were tokened and Premacked. No strategy was successful in raising performance level of these behaviors to a high level except the Premack contingencies alone, which resulted in a final performance level near 100 percent.

SUBJECT 29

Presenting Problems

Subject 29 (R.L.) is a thirteen-year-old white male of low average intelligence. He was referred for treatment primarily because of behavior problems while residing at a psychiatric ward of a state hospital. He had come to this hopsital two years earlier from an institutional home for boys.

The immediate presenting behavior problems were foul language, hyperactivity, frequent runaways, stealing, lying, extreme verbal aggression, and hospitality. In addition, there was a background of homosexual activity.

Cottage and School Programs

R.L. was admitted for treatment on January 5, 1970. Goals of the cottage program were to have him take more responsibility for himself, to help him set up reasonable goals for his life, and to help him to handle his behavior problems, such as stealing, lying, and running away.

His Level I program designated the following categories of behavior as targets:

Interaction—20 marks   PE behavior—3 marks
Physical contact—20 marks   Self-help skills—5 marks
General compliance—15 marks School—25 marks

On Level II, the targets were as follows:

Improving social skills—20 marks   Self-help skills—12 marks
Compliance—5 marks   Job (Put away cottage
Special sessions—5 marks   bikes—0 marks
Table manners—15 marks   School—20 marks

He was placed on the time-out punishment condition.

Data

Independent Observations

There was a clear increase in the extent to which R.L. engaged in positive interactions with peers on the unit. During the first four weeks of treatment, such behavior accounted for the following percentages of all unit observations: 1.5, 4.0, 10.7, and 9.9, respectively. The corresponding figures for the four weeks immediately preceding the end of the project were 28.9 percent, 42.0 percent, 41.1 percent, and 40.8 percent. Other unit measures, such as the percentage deviant index, did not show any clear trend to the present time.

The percentage deviant index for the school observations remained low (below 6%), with the exceptions of the first week in school and the tenth week of school (8.5%). There were no clear trends in any of the other school measures.

Daily Checklist

Beginning in January, the behaviors that had both tokened and Premacked contingencies were room neat, closets and drawers neat, brushing teeth after lunch and dinner, and showers. At the end of April, the additional behaviors that were tokened and Premacked included bed made, hair neat, dressed neat, brush teeth at breakfast laundry, and in room on time at night. Also there were token contingencies for good manners at all meals. Between January and April, the four behaviors that were initially connected with contingencies increased steadily in frequency, from the rate of 46.6 percent the first week to 100 percent for the last week in April. After the addition of the other contingencies, neither these behaviors nor the newly tokened behaviors were performed at such a high rate. The aggregate level of performance of check list behaviors with contingencies averaged around 70 percent, with a great deal of variability.

SUBJECT 30

Presenting Problems

Subject 30 (D.G.) is an eleven-year-old white male, who is functionally retarded. He was referred for treatment because of stealing behavior at home and at school.

His family consisted only of a mother. There was reportedly

inappropriate intimacy between mother and son, including sleeping together and body fondling.

D.G. engaged in stealing both from his mother and at school. At school, he had very poor peer relationships and reportedly provoked black children. Academically, he was functioning at a very low, preprimer level.

Cottage and School Programs

D.G. was admitted to the cottage on February 2, 1970.

On his Level I program (70 tokens possible), the categories of behavior designated as targets were being with older kids, accepting adult decisions, masculine activities, generally appropriate social behavior, MABs (room neat, closets and drawers, brushing teeth).

After two weeks on baseline, D.G. was placed on the response-cost punishment condition. Response cost proved highly successful in reducing the frequency of deviant behavior from baseline.

Data

Independent Observations

During 13 weeks, percent deviant behavior declined from 17.1 percent the first week to 0.8 percent the last. Increases over time in positive interaction with peers and decreases in negative verbalizations were tentative trends in the data. Percent deviant in school did not exceed 5 percent at the end of the project.

Daily Checklist

Minimal acceptable behaviors tokened were room neat, closets and drawers neat, and brushing teeth after all three meals. Performance of tokened behaviors the first three weeks was 55, 63, and 77 percent respectively, and for the last three weeks, 89, 89, and 96 percent. The nontokened behaviors were performed steadily around the 90 percent level.

Appendix F

SAMPLES OF INSTRUMENTS USED IN FOLLOW-UP STUDY

Appendix F provides samples of the instruments used in the follow-up study that was done for the research project. The instruments are arranged, with the appendix, in the following order:

1. Parent Questionnaire
2. School Questionnaire
3. Follow-up Rating Form

PARENT QUESTIONNAIRE

Part I　　　　　　　　　　　　Yes Sometimes No　*Is this a big problem?*

1. Does the child dress himself?
2. Does the child wash his hands?
3. Does the child use good table manners?
4. Does the child take a shower or bath often enough?
5. Does the child brush his teeth often enough?
6. Is the child usually on time to things such as meals and school?
7. Does the child use the toilet properly?
8. Does the child wet or soil his bed or pants?

Comments:

Part II　　　　　　　　　　Never　*Some-times*　*Fre-quently*　*Is this a big problem?*

1. Does the child fail to things that you have often told him to do?
2. Does the child do expected household chores?
3. Does the child do things that you have told him again and again he should not do?
4. Is the child sassy or disrespectful to adults?
5. Does the child refuse to help other people when he is asked to help?
6. When the child is upset,

Appendix F 275

| | *Never* | *Some-times* | *Fre-quently* | *Is this a big problem?* |

Part II

does he hit, kick, or bite other people?
7. Does the child take things that do not belong to him?
8. Does the child try to tease or provoke other children?
9. Does the child refuse to share his things with others when he should share them?
10. Does the child tear up things which do not belong to him?
11. Does the child use curse words?
12. Does the child tell lies?
13. Does the child cheat at games?
14. Does the child throw tantrums or temper fits?
15. Does the child tear up his own things?
16. Does the child try to hurt himself in any way, for instance biting himself, hitting his head on tables or walls, or any other way?
17. Does the child participate in group games with other children?
18. Does the child talk with other people?
19. When the child talks, do his sentences make sense?
20. Does the child talk too loud?

	Never	Some-times	Fre-quently	Is this a big problem?

21. Does the child play with other children?
22. Is the child too silly?
23. Does the child laugh for long periods of time when there seems to be no good reason for laughing?
24. Does the child cry for long periods of time when there seems to be no good reason for being sad?
25. Does the child complain about physical ailments?
26. Has the child been in trouble with the law?
27. Does the child masturbate?
28. If the child is a boy, is he too feminine; or if the child is a girl, is she too masculine?
29. Has the child made any sexual assaults?

Comments:

Part III

1. Are there any outstanding problems with this child?   If so, please describe them.

2. How does the child get along with his brothers and sisters?

Appendix F

3. How does the child get along with you?

4. Is the child behaving any differently since his stay at Adler? If so, please describe how — both behaviors that are better and those that are worse.

5. Is the child still receiving professional help?   Where?

SCHOOL QUESTIONNAIRE

Part I
1. About how many days of school per month does the child miss school?
2. About how many days per month is the child late to school?
3. What is the child's average school mark?
4. What is the child's average conduct grade in school?

	Never	Not very often	Frequently	Is this a problem?	Does not apply

Part II
1. In school, is the child often out of his seat without permission?
2. Does the child ignore spoken or written instructions in school and appear to just "not pay attention"?
3. Does the child answer questions in class?

	Never	Not very often	Fre- quently	Is this a problem?	Does not apply

4. Does the child make "catcalls" or any other noises to try to disrupt the teacher or the class in school?
5. In school, does the child try to distract other children from their work?
6. Does the child throw objects at other people?
7. Does the child physically assault other children?
8. Does the child make threats to other people to try to get his own way?
9. Does the child have a "quick temper" — does he "fly off the handle" easily?
10. Does the child use profanity?
11. Does the child comply with requests made by adults?
12. Is the child sassy or disrespectful to adults?
13. Does the child refuse to help others when he is asked to help?
14. Does the child refuse to share his things with others?
15. Does the child steal?
16. Is the child destructive?
17. Does the child tell lies?
18. Does the child cheat at games?

Appendix F 279

| | Never | Not very often | Fre- quently | Is this a problem? | Does not apply |

19. Is the child self-destructive?
20. Does the child talk with other people?
21. When the child talks, do his sentences make sense?
22. Does the child complain about physical ailments?
23. Does the child masturbate in class?
24. Does the child complete work designed to do during class?
25. Does the child complete homework assignments?

Part III

1. Are there any outstanding problems with this child? If so, please state them specifically.

2. Is the child behaving any differently since his stay at Adler? If so, please specify both the behaviors that are better and those that are worse.

FOLLOW-UP RATING FORM

No.

At the present time what is the status of the presenting problems which precipitated admission to Adler?

1. The problem behavior is present and appears more serious (higher frequency, duration, and intensity or combination thereof) than before.
2. The problem remains at a level of seriousness comparable to that prior to admission (same frequency, duration, and intensity).
3. The problem behavior remains, but at a less serious level than

that prior to admission (reduced frequency, intensity, and duration).

4. The problem behavior is present but at an intensity, frequency, and duration which is to be expected of the normal population.

Family:	School:
1.	1.
2.	2.
3.	3.
4.	4.
5.	5.
Personal:	Neighborhood:
1.	1.
2.	2.
3.	3.

What is the status of the present problems which are not part of the summary of presenting problems? i.e. those listed under Present Problems Not Similar to Those Prior to Admission?

1. The problem merits the intervention of professions at the level of residential treatment.

2. The problem merits outpatient services of a long term nature (10 or more weekly sessions).

3. The problem merits short term outpatient services (5 to 10 weekly sessions).

4. The problem can be alleviated by limited consultation with parents or teacher.

5. The problem is such that it can be handled easily by the parents or teacher and requires no intervention by professionals.

Of what significance do you feel the reports of the perceived progress to be?

1. The types of behavior reported are those that will contribute significantly to the child's meeting of societal demands in the areas of prosocial behavior in the home and/or in the classroom.

2. The types of behavior reported are those that will contribute in a small way to the child's meeting of societal demands in the areas of prosocial behavior in the home and in the classroom.

3. The types of behaviors reported are likely to improve significantly the child's relationships with adults (teachers and parents) who maintain guardian type roles in home and school.
4. The types of behaviors reported are likely to improve to a small degree the child's relationships with adults (teachers and parents) who maintain guardian type roles in the home and school.
5. The types of behavior reported are likely to make the child more likeable to his peer group.
6. None of the behaviors reported under this heading are clinically significant or important with respect to improvement.

INDEX

A

Adler Zone Center, Herman M., 3, 50, 62, 71
  administration, 7-9
  admission procedures, 9-10
  Clinical Review Committee, 10, 62
  goals of, 5
  gym, 4, 62
  map of, 4
  organizational chart, 8
  school, 4, 62, 76-77, 78-81
  staff, 7-9
  Superintendent, 7, 8
Appropriate social behaviors (ASB)
  categories of, 17-18
  constructive, 18, 36, 126
  cooperation, 17, 36, 126
  definition of, 17
  of Dimension 3, 17-18
  helping, 18, 36, 126
  individual programs
    Subject 1, 222-23, 224
    Subject 2, 225-26
    Subject 3, 227-28, 229
    Subject 4, 229-30
    Subject 5, 231-32, 233
    Subject 6, 234-35
    Subject 7, 237, 238
    Subject 8, 239-40
    Subject 9, 241
    Subject 10, 85, 86, 87
    Subject 11, 243
    Subject 12, 245
    Subject 13, 246-47
    Subject 14, 248
    Subject 15, 250
    Subject 16, 252
    Subject 17, 253
    Subject 18, 255
    Subject 19, 91-92, 93, 94, 95
    Subject 20, 257
    Subject 21, 102, 103-05
    Subject 22, 258
    Subject 23, 259
    Subject 24, 261
    Subject 25, 263-64
    Subject 26, 265-66
    Subject 27, 267
    Subject 28, 269
    Subject 29, 270
    Subject 30, 272
  interaction, 18, 36, 126
  participation, 18, 36, 126
  sharing, 18, 36, 126
  and training staff, 54-55
  see also Dimension 3
ASB, *see* Appropriate social behaviors

B

Backups, *see* Reinforcers, program of

C

Cardex, 65
  sample of, 199-202, 204-08, 210-13, 218
Child
  data book on, 42-43, 66-67
  home visits for, 81
  log book on, 66
  opportunities for
    cooperation, 36
    helping, 36
    constructive behavior, 36
    interaction, 36
    participation, 36
    sharing, 36
  program as guideline to staff, 71
  relationship to others
    community, 50, 51
    family, 51
    staff, 60-61
  and treatment process, 33-37
    coping capacity defined, 35

coping patterns defined, 35
program altered when, 36-37
program set up for each child, 35-37
notion of adaptation, 36
notion of creativity, 36
respect for child in, 33-34
teach child to respect others, 34
Child-care staff, *see* Staff positions
Children's Research Center, 3, 50, 51
administration, 7-9
Director, 7, 8
goals of, 5-6
map of, 4
organizational chart, 8
staff, 7-9
Clinical Review Committee, 10, 62
Communication, *see* Staff communication
Coping capacity, 35
Coping patterns
and altering child's program, 37
defined, 35
Cottage Director, 7, 8, 10, 63, 69
duties and responsibilities, 140-41
Cottage G, 3
admission criteria for, 10
description of, 62
floor plan of, 63
length of child's stay in, 10, 62
personnel, 7
Cottage program, 67-78
daily schedule, 76-78
feedback and reinforcement, 71-74
levels of, 67-71
Level I, 69-70
Level II, 70
Level III, 70-71
Orientation Level, 67-69
punishment, 74-76
response cost, 75-76
time out, 74-75
treatment planning meetings, 68-69, 70
see also Cottage and school programs
Cottage and school programs
individual programs
Subject 1, 222-23
Subject 2, 225-26
Subject 3, 227-28
Subject 4, 229-30
Subject 5, 231-32
Subject 6, 234-35
Subject 7, 237
Subject 8, 239-40
Subject 9, 241
Subject 10, 85-87
Subject 11, 243-44
Subject 12, 245
Subject 13, 246-47
Subject 14, 248
Subject 15, 249-50
Subject 16, 252
Subject 17, 253
Subject 18, 255
Subject 19, 90-95
Subject 20, 256-57
Subject 21, 102-06
Subject 22, 258
Subject 23, 259-60
Subject 24, 261
Subject 25, 263-64
Subject 26, 265-66
Subject 27, 267
Subject 28, 269
Subject 29, 270
Subject 30, 272

D

Daily Checklist, 38, 39-41
data analysis of, 39-41
subdivision of items, 39
use of computer in, 39
of Dimension 2, 16-17
list of items on, 40
as MAB performance measure, 39-41
Orientation Level and, 39-40, 68
reliability of, 39-40
checks on, 39
data on, 39-41
table of overall, 40
as research instrument, 16-17, 39-41
sample instrument, 146
Subject 9, 242
Subject 10, 89
Subject 11, 244

Subject 12, 246
Subject 13, 247
Subject 14, 249
Subject 15, 251
Subject 16, 252-53
Subject 17, 254
Subject 18, 256
Subject 19, 99-100
Subject 20, 257
Subject 21, 109-10
Subject 22, 259
Subject 23, 260
Subject 25, 264
Subject 26, 266
Subject 27, 268
Subject 28, 269-70
Subject 29, 271
Subject 30, 272
use of, 39
see also Dimension 2, Minimum appropriate behaviors
Daily Schedule of Activities, 57
  implementation of, 76-78
  procedures and policies, 178-81
Data, *see* Daily Checklist, Independent Observations, Punishment data
Dimension 1, 14-16
  assessment of, 125
  in cottage program, 67-71
  definition of, 13
  as guideline, 13-14
  evolvement of, 21-22
  Level I of, 15-16
  Level II of, 16
    phases identified in, 16
  Level III of, 16
  Orientation Level of, 15
    use of Daily Checklist on, 39-41
  and training staff, 53-54
  and treatment process, 35
  use of Mark Sheet in, 19
  see also Level I, Level II, Level III, Mark Sheet, Orientation Level
Dimension 2, 16-17
  assessment of, 125-26
  and cottage program, 71-74
  Daily Checklist, 16-17, 39-41
  definition of, 13

evolvement of, 22-23
  as guideline, 13-14
  minimum appropriate behaviors, 16-17
  and training staff, 54
  and treatment process, 35-36
  see also Daily Checklist, Minimum appropriate behaviors
Dimension 3, 17-18
  appropriate social behavior categories, 17-18
    constructive, 18, 36
    cooperation, 17, 36
    helping, 18, 36
    interaction, 18, 36
    participation, 18, 36
    sharing, 17, 36
  assessment of, 126-27
  and cottage program, 71-74
  definition of, 13
  evolvement of, 22-23
  as guideline, 14
  Independent Observations, 44-48
  and training staff, 54-55
  and treatment process, 35-36
  see also Appropriate social behaviors
Dimension 4, 18-20
  assessment of, 127
  in cottage program, 71-74
  definition of, 13
  evolvement of, 26-29
    relation to other dimensions, 30-31
  feedback system of, 18-19
  as guideline, 14
  Mark Sheet, 19, 41-43
  program of reinforcers, 19-20
    backup, 19-20
    social, 19-20
  and training staff, 55
  and treatment process, 35
  see also Feedback system, Mark Sheet, Reinforcers, program of
Dimension 5, 20-21
  assessment of, 128
  categories of punishable behavior, 20-21
    100-700 Level list, 20
  in cottage program, 74-76

definition of, 13
evolvement of, 24-26
  relation to other dimensions, 31-32
as guideline, 14
punishment study, 113-24
punishment system of, 20-21
response-cost procedure and, 20
time-out procedure and, 20
and training staff, 55-56
and treatment process, 35, 36
see also Punishment system, Response cost, Time out

Dimensions
assessment of, 125-28
definition of, 13
evolvement of, 21-32
as guidelines, 13-14
as guidelines for child, 37
of the milieu, 13-32
see also Dimension 1, Dimension 2, Dimension 3, Dimension 4, Dimension 5

E
Extramural Case Coordinator, 7, 8, 10, 38, 41, 50, 52, 56, 64-66, 69, 80-82
duties and responsibilities of, 141

F
Feedback system
  cottage program and, 71-74
  of Dimension 4, 18-19
  Mark Sheet use in, 19
  see also Dimension 4, Mark Sheet
500 Level behaviors
  list of, 21
  see also Dimension 5
Follow-up study
  instruments for
    Parent Questionnaire, 129-30, 274-77
    Rating Form, 131-32, 279-81
    School Questionnaire, 129-30, 277-79
  pilot study, 129-34
    analyses of data, 131-33
    description of sample, 130-31
400 Level behaviors
  list of, 21
  see also Dimension 5

H
Home program, 81-83
  child's home visits, 81
  family and staff relationship, 81-82
  implementation problems, 82-83
  related to cottage program, 82
  Subject 10, 87-88
  Subject 14, 248-49
  Subject 19, 95-96
  Subject 21, 106
  Subject 27, 267
Home visit forms, sample of, 219-20

I
Illinois Department of Mental Health, 3, 7
Independent Observations, 38, 44-48
  categories and classification of behavior, 45-46
  cottage
    Subject 1, 223
    Subject 2, 226
    Subject 3, 228
    Subject 4, 230
    Subject 5, 232-33
    Subject 6, 235
    Subject 7, 237
    Subject 8, 240
    Subject 9, 241-42
    Subject 10, 88
    Subject 11, 244
    Subject 12, 245-46
    Subject 13, 247
    Subject 14, 249
    Subject 15, 251
    Subject 16, 252
    Subject 17, 254
    Subject 18, 256
    Subject 19, 96-97
    Subject 20, 257
    Subject 21, 106-09
    Subject 22, 258
    Subject 23, 260
    Subject 24, 261-62
    Subject 25, 264
    Subject 26, 266
    Subject 27, 268
    Subject 28, 269

Subject 29, 270-71
Subject 30, 272
description of observational instrument, 45
  schematic representation of classifications, 45
Dimension 3, 45
Independent Observations Handbook, 45, 46
  sample of, 160-69
made when and where, 44-45, 46
Observer's Rating Sheet, 46, 170
Observer's Summary Sheet, 46, 171
procedure for, 44-46
rating behaviors, 46
reliability of, 46-48
  data for, 47
school
  Subject 1, 223-24
  Subject 2, 226
  Subject 3, 228
  Subject 4, 230
  Subject 5, 233
  Subject 6, 235
  Subject 7, 237-38
  Subject 8, 240
  Subject 9, 241-42
  Subject 10, 89
  Subject 11, 244
  Subject 12, 245-46
  Subject 13, 247
  Subject 14, 249
  Subject 15, 251
  Subject 16, 252
  Subject 17, 254
  Subject 18, 256
  Subject 19, 97-99
  Subject 20, 257
  Subject 21, 108-09
  Subject 22, 258
  Subject 23, 260
  Subject 24, 262
  Subject 25, 264
  Subject 27, 268
  Subject 28, 269
  Subject 29, 271
  Subject 30, 272
staff described, 44

use of data, 47-48
see also **Dimension 3**
Independent Observations Handbook, 45, 46
  sample of, 160-67
    examples of categorized behaviors, 167-69
Individual programs
  Subject 1, 222-24
  Subject 2, 224-27
  Subject 3, 227-29
  Subject 4, 229-30
  Subject 5, 231-34
  Subject 6, 234-36
  Subject 7, 236-38
  Subject 8, 238-40
  Subject 9, 241-42
  Subject 10, 84-90
  Subject 11, 242-44
  Subject 12, 244-46
  Subject 13, 246-47
  Subject 14, 247-49
  Subject 15, 249-51
  Subject 16, 251-53
  Subject 17, 253-54
  Subject 18, 254-56
  Subject 19, 90-101, 197-220
  Subject 20, 256-57
  Subject 21, 101-12
  Subject 22, 257-59
  Subject 23, 259-60
  Subject 24, 260-62
  Subject 25, 263-64
  Subject 26, 264-66
  Subject 27, 266-68
  Subject 28, 268-70
  Subject 29, 270-71
  Subject 30, 271-72
  see also Cottage and school programs, Home program, Presenting problems
Instruments for evaluation, 38-49
  Daily Checklist, 39-41
    analyzed how, 39-41
    sample of, 146
  data processing 38
  Independent Observations, 44-48
    sample of handbook, 160-69

288   *A Milieu Therapy Program for Disturbed Children*

    sample of Observer's Rating Sheet, 170
    sample of Observer's Summary Sheet, 171
  list of, 38
  Mark Sheet, 41-43
    sample of, 147-49
  other instruments, 48-49
    Behavior Description Form, 48
    Rating Checklist, 49
    token earning, 48
  Special Behavior Report Form, 43-44
    analyzed how, 43-44
    samples of, 154, 158, 159
  see also Daily Checklist, Independent Observations, Mark Sheet, Special Behavior Report Form
Instruments for follow-up study
  Parent Questionnaire
    sample of, 274-77
  Rating Form
    sample of, 279-81
  School Questionnaire
    sample of, 277-79
Intramural Counselor, 7, 8, 41, 43, 50, 58
  and communication channels, 64-67
  and cottage program, 68-70, 73
  duties and responsibilities of, 141-43
  and home program, 81-83
  and program planning, 62-64
  and school planning, 78-81

L

Level I
  cardex sample for, 199-202
  in cottage program, 69-70
  of Dimension 1, 15-16
  Mark Sheet, 19
    example of completed, 198
  Subject 9, 241
  Subject 10, 85-86
  Subject 11, 243
  Subject 12, 245
  Subject 13, 246
  Subject 16, 252
  Subject 17, 253
  Subject 18, 255

  Subject 19, 91
  Subject 20, 256-57
  Subject 21, 102-03
  Subject 22, 258
  Subject 23, 259
  Subject 24, 261
  Subject 25, 263
  Subject 26, 265
  Subject 27, 267
  Subject 28, 269
  Subject 29, 270
  Subject 30, 272
  see also Appropriate social behaviors, Dimension 1, Minimum appropriate behaviors, Punishment contingency
Level II
  cardex samples for, 204-08, 210-13, 215-17
  in cottage program, 70
  of Dimension 1, 16
  Mark Sheet example, 203, 209, 214
  Phases I-IV of, 16
  Subject 9, 241
  Subject 10, 86-87
  Subject 11, 243
  Subject 12, 245
  Subject 13, 246
  Subject 17, 253
  Subject 18, 255
  Subject 19, 91-95
  Subject 20, 257
  Subject 21, 103-06
  Subject 22, 258
  Subject 23, 259-60
  Subject 24, 261
  Subject 25, 264
  Subject 26, 266
  Subject 27, 267
  Subject 28, 269
  Subject 29, 270
  see also Appropriate social behaviors, Dimension 1, Minimum appropriate behaviors, Punishment contingency
Level III
  cardex sample for, 218
  in cottage program, 70-71
  of Dimension 1, 16

Subject 9, 241
Subject 13, 247
Subject 18, 255
Subject 19, 95
see also Appropriate social behaviors, Dimension 1, Minimum appropriate behaviors, Punishment contingency

M

MAB, see Minimum appropriate behaviors
Mark Sheet, 19, 38, 41-43
  and cottage program, 67-74
  data on, 42
    recorded in child's data book, 42
  description of, 41-42
  example of completed, 198, 203, 209, 214
  implementation of, 71-74
  kinds of, 42
    response cost, 42
    school, 42, 79
    time out, 42
  sample instrument
    response cost, 148
    school, 149
    time out, 147
  and school program, 78-80
  used daily as record of
    child's achievement, 42
    child's target behaviors, 42
    difficulty of child's program, 42-43
    marks earned and spent, 42
    staff attitude toward child, 42-43
    staff giving marks, 42
  see also Dimension 4, Feedback system
Milieu, of research project, 12-32
Milieu program
  communication channels, 64-67
  cottage program, 67-78
  home program, 81-83
  implementation of, 62-83
  planning, 62-64
  school program, 78-81
  see also Cottage program, Home program, School program
Milieu therapy, definition of, 12
Minimum appropriate behaviors (MABs)
  Daily Checklist of, 39-41
    sample of, 146
  of Dimension 2, 16-17
  individual programs
    Subject 1, 224
    Subject 2, 226-27
    Subject 3, 229
    Subject 4, 230
    Subject 5, 231-32, 233-34
    Subject 6, 236
    Subject 7, 238
    Subject 8, 240
    Subject 9, 241
    Subject 10, 85, 86, 87
    Subject 11, 243
    Subject 12, 245
    Subject 13, 246-47
    Subject 14, 248
    Subject 15, 250
    Subject 17, 253
    Subject 18, 255
    Subject 19, 91, 92, 93, 94, 95
    Subject 20, 257
    Subject 21, 102-03, 104, 105
    Subject 22, 258
    Subject 24, 261
    Subject 25, 263-64
    Subject 26, 265
    Subject 27, 267
    Subject 28, 269
    Subject 29, 270
    Subject 30, 272
  and training for staff, 54
  see also Daily Checklist, Dimension 2

O

Observer's Rating Sheet
  Independent Observations, 46
  sample of, 170
Observer's Summary Sheet
  Independent Observations, 46
  sample of, 171
100 Level behaviors
  list of, 20
  see also Dimension 5
Organizational chart, of research project, 8
Orientation Level

in cottage program, 67-69
of Dimension 1, 15
procedures and policies, 174-78
   data recording, 174-75
   general, 177
   home visits, 176
   Mark Sheet lost, 177
   off-unit activities, 176
   prices, 176
   punishment, 175-76
   specific, 178
   treats, 177
and punishment study, 113-24
and treatment process, 35
use of Daily Checklist on, 39-40
use of Special Behavior Report Form on, 43
see also Dimension 1

P

Phases I-IV, see Level II
Premack principle, 29, 41, 53-54, 70, 82
   in individual programs, 99-100, 110, 246, 250, 254, 255, 269-70, 271
Presenting problems
   Subject 1, 222
   Subject 2, 224-25
   Subject 3, 227
   Subject 4, 229
   Subject 5, 231
   Subject 6, 234
   Subject 7, 236
   Subject 8, 238-39
   Subject 9, 241
   Subject 10, 84
   Subject 11, 242-43
   Subject 12, 244-45
   Subject 13, 246
   Subject 14, 247-48
   Subject 15, 249
   Subject 16, 251-52
   Subject 17, 253
   Subject 18, 254-55
   Subject 19, 90
   Subject 20, 256
   Subject 21, 101-02
   Subject 22, 257-58
   Subject 23, 259

   Subject 24, 260-61
   Subject 25, 263
   Subject 26, 264-65
   Subject 27, 266-67
   Subject 28, 268-69
   Subject 29, 270
   Subject 30, 271-72
Program
   milieu, 62-83
   planning, 62-64
   see also Cottage program, Cottage and school program, Home program, School program
Project Coordinator, 7, 8, 9, 10, 63-64, 69
   duties and responsibilities of, 140
Project Director, 7, 8, 10, 63-64, 65, 69
Punishment contingency
and cottage program, 69-70, 74-76
procedures and policies, 182-91
   100 Level, 182-84
   200 Level, 184-86
   300 Level, 186-89
   400 Level, 189-90
   500 Level, 190
   600 Level, 191
   700 Level, 191
and school program, 79
Subject 9, 118
Subject 10, 85, 86, 87, 118
Subject 11, 243-44
Subject 12, 118, 120
Subject 13, 118, 120
Subject 14, 118, 248
Subject 15, 118
Subject 16, 118
Subject 17, 118, 120
Subject 18, 118
Subject 19, 91, 92, 93, 94, 95, 118
Subject 20, 118
Subject 21, 103, 104, 105, 118, 120
Subject 22, 258
Subject 23, 118, 261
Subject 24, 118, 264
Subject 25, 118, 120, 266
Subject 26, 118
Subject 27, 118, 120
Subject 28, 118

Subject 29, 270
Subject 30, 272
see also Response cost, Time out
Punishment data
  Subject 10, 89-90
  Subject 19, 100-01
  Subject 21, 110-12
Punishment study, 113-24
  discussion, 121-24
  results, 115-20
    across all subjects, 115-17
    on individual subjects, 120
    between the two groups, 117-19
    within the two groups, 119-20
  Special Behavior Report Form, 43-44
  summary, 124
Punishment system
  categories of behavior, 20-21
  and cottage program, 74-76
  of Dimension 5, 20-21
  response cost, 20-21
  time out, 20-21
  and training staff to use, 55-56
  and treatment process, 36
  see also Dimension 5, Response cost, Time out

R

Reinforcers, program of
  backups, 19-20
    in cottage program, 67-74
    list of, 181-82
  cottage program and, 67-74
  of Dimension 4, 19-20
  Mark Sheet used in, 42
  social, 19-20
  and training staff, 55
  see also Dimension 4
Research project
  administration of, 7-9
  admission to cottage, 9-10
  assessment of, 125-34
    conceptualization and implementation, 125-29
    outcome, 129
    pilot follow-up study, 129-33
    summary, 133-34
  framework of, 11

goals of, 6
milieu of, 12-32
organizational chart, 8
procedures and policies
  backups, list of, 181-82
  Daily Schedule of Activities, 178-81
  Orientation Level, 174-78
  punishment contingencies, 182-91
  response cost, 193-95
  time out, 191-93
Project Director, 7, 8, 10
sample, 10-11
staff, 7-9
  and implementation of milieu program, 62-83
see also Cottage G, Staff positions
Response cost
  child assigned randomly to, 70
  and cottage program, 74-76
  Dimension 5 and, 20
  earning power per day on, 76
  list of penalties, 76
  Mark Sheet used in, 42
  procedures, 193-95
    recording and payment of fines, 195
  in punishment study, 113-24
  in punishment system, 20-21
  Special Behavior Report Form, 43-44
  see also Dimension 5, Punishment system

S

School program, 78-81
  public school, 80
  see also Cottage and school program
700 Level behaviors
  list of, 21
  see also Dimension 5
600 Level behaviors
  list of, 21
  see also Dimension 5
Special Behavior Report Form, 38, 43-44
  data analysis of, 43-44
    child's acceptance of punishment, 44
    in punishment study, 43-44, 113-24
    recorded in child's data book, 43

staff distribution of invoked contingencies, 44
use of computer in, 43
description of, 43
information provided by, 43-44
instructions for completion of, 150-53, 155-57
kinds of, 43
  baseline, 43
  response cost, 43
  time out, 43
Orientation Level and, 43
sample instrument
  baseline, 159
  response cost, 158
  time out, 154
see also Dimension 5, Punishment study
Staff communication, 64-67
cardex, 65
child's data book, 66-67
child's log book, 66
meetings, 64-65
memory aids, 66
report book, 66
staff slips, 65-66
Staff positions
Assistant Counselor, 7
Child Care Aide, 7
Cottage Director, 7, 8, 10, 140-41
Extramural Case Coordinator, 7, 8, 10, 38, 41, 50, 52, 56, 64-66, 69, 80-82, 141
Independent Observers, 7, 8, 44
Intramural Counselor, 7, 8, 41, 43, 50, 58
  and communication channels, 64-67
  and cottage program, 68-70, 73
  duties and responsibilities of, 141-43
  and home program, 81-83
  and program planning, 62-64
  and school planning, 78-81
Mental Health Program Assistant, 7
Mental Health Worker, 7
Program Director, Adler, 8, 10
Project Coordinator, 7, 8, 9, 10, 63-64, 69, 140

Project Director, 7, 8, 10, 63-64, 65, 69
Project Secretary, 7, 8
research assistants, 7, 8
school teacher, Adler, 10, 38, 64, 65, 78
school teacher, public, 65, 80
Subject 1, 133, 222-24
Subject 2, 133, 224-27
Subject 3, 133, 227-29
Subject 4, 133, 229-30
Subject 5, 133, 231-34
Subject 6, 133, 234-36
Subject 7, 133, 236-38
Subject 8, 133, 238-40
Subject 9, 118, 133, 241-42
Subject 10, 84-90, 118, 133
Subject 11, 133, 242-44
Subject 12, 118, 120, 244-46
Subject 13, 118, 120, 133, 246-47
Subject 14, 118, 133, 247-49
Subject 15, 118, 133, 249-51
Subject 16, 118, 251-53
Subject 17, 118, 120, 253-54
Subject 18, 118, 133, 254-56
Subject 19, 90-101, 118, 133, 197-220
Subject 20, 118, 133, 256-57
Subject 21, 101-12, 118, 120
Subject 22, 133, 257-59
Subject 23, 118, 259-60
Subject 24, 118, 260-62
Subject 25, 118, 120, 263-64
Subject 26, 118, 264-66
Subject 27, 118, 120, 266-68
Subject 28, 118, 268-70
Subject 29, 270-71
Subject 30, 271-72

T

Target behaviors, 69-70
  see also Appropriate social behaviors, Minimum appropriate behaviors
Time out
  child assigned randomly to, 70
  and cottage program, 74-75
  description of room used for, 74
  Dimension 5 and, 20
  list of penalties, 76

procedures, 191-93
  cottage, 192-93
  school, 191-92
in punishment study, 113-24
in punishment system, 20-21
and school program, 79
Special Behavior Report Form, 43-44
see also Dimension 5, Punishment system
300 Level behaviors
list of, 20-21
see also Dimension 5
Training for staff, 50-61
  areas considered in, 50-52
    Adler Zone Center, 50-51
    Children's Research Center, 50, 51-52
    individual child's family, 50, 51
    other agencies including foster homes, 50, 51
  basic concept of, 52
  cottage management, 56-57
    allocation of time in, 56-57
    communication in, 56
    schedule of daily activities for, 57
  dimensions of the milieu, 52-56
    Dimension 1, 53-54
    Dimension 2, 54
    Dimension 3, 54-55
    Dimension 4, 55
    Dimension 5, 55-56
  individual child care, 60-61
    crisis situations, methods for dealing with, 60-61
    preparation of detailed daily schedule for, 60
    techniques of interviewing, 61
  length of, 50
  list of program areas, 52
  observation and recording, 59-60
    collecting and displaying of data, 59
    forms used by cottage staff, 58-59
    intrepretation of specific behavior, 60
    three-term contingency (ABC) introduced, 59
  physical health and drugs, 58-59
    administering drugs to a child, 59
    common pediatric illnesses, 58-59
    problem of physical illness, 59
    relationship of child-care staff and nursing and medical staff, 58
  recreation and arts and crafts activities, 57-58
    allocation of time for, 57
    kinds of, 57
    relationship of child to group activities, 57-58
  school and cottage coordination, 58
    relationship of child-care worker's role and teacher's role, 58
    techniques and problems in, 58
  summary, 61
    involvement of staff in ongoing training, 61
    need for continuous training, 61
    staff member as initiator, 61
  teaching methods used
    discussion, 50, 52
    lecture, 50
    role playing, 50, 52
    written exercises, 50
200 Level behaviors
list of, 20
see also Dimension 5

U

University of Illinois, 3, 7, 44
  Digital Computer Laboratory, 38

Date Due

| MAR 1 3 '74 | | | |